VIBRANT HAPPY YOU

CLARA V.
RODRIGUEZ

Vibrant Happy You:
7 Simple Solutions to Relieve Anxiety and Depression
By Clara V. Rodriguez, M.A. RYT 200

Published by Ananda Total Wellbeing, LLC
Copyright 2018 by Clara V. Rodriguez
All rights reserved
ISBN-13: 978-1-7327734-1-7
Illustrations by Ilana Cloud
Cover Photo by Samantha Castillo

Important Legal Notice and Disclaimer

This publication is intended to provide educational information with regard to the subject matter covered.

The reader of this book assumes all responsibility for the use of this information. The author and Ananda Total Wellbeing, LLC assume no responsibility or liability whatsoever on behalf of any purchaser or reader of these materials. The methodology and teaching do not guarantee success, and results may vary.

The author of this book does not provide psychological or medical advice nor prescribe the use of any technique as a form of treatment. This book is not intended to heal, cure, or advise nor prescribe the use of any treatment for any type of mental or physical health issues or otherwise. Before attempting any of the physical movements or exercises, please see your physician to ensure you are in the right condition to pursue the exercise(s).

TABLE OF CONTENTS

DEDICATION

This book is dedicated to the two biggest miracles in my life – my nephew and my niece, so that they might grow up in a generous, loving world full of acceptance, peace, and happiness.

This book is also dedicated to my loving parents and my first teachers. To my dad, for being my first mentor on how to share my gifts with the world through education and writing. May you live on in the difference you taught me to make in the world through this book and all the lives it touches. To my mom, who continues to show me on a daily basis how to take things in stride and live generously. Thank you, mom, for your immense support, dedication, and love. Te amo.

This book is also dedicated to my sisters for helping me make it through the tough years of my journey before I had these tools. For loving and forgiving me when I didn't know how to truly love and forgive. For being my best friends now and people I can count on. I love you.

GRATITUDE LIST

I am grateful to all the teachers, coaches, mentors, friends and acquaintances who have guided me, supported me and loved me throughout this journey. All that I am able to give to the world is because of all that I have lived and learned, thanks to you.

I am forever grateful to my book coach, Lenear Bassett-King, for her unwavering commitment to keeping me in action and getting this book out to the world. A very special thanks to my editors and partners in creativity, Cheryl McCoy, Melissa Pauls and Sarah Gingrich; without whose brilliance and finesse this book would not have the clarity and flow to make the difference. A huge acknowledgement to my yoga mentors, Sara Vandergoot and Deborah Jackson, my illustrator, Ilana Cloud, my photographer, Samantha Castillo, and my business mentor, Debbie Orol. To all my mentors, coaches and teammates that contributed to my amazing journey of growth and expansion, thank you.

A huge hug to my loving and inspirational friends, Ayda Nesvaderani, Daphne Erhart and Martie Pineda for their contributions, support and inspiration that made this book possible.

FOREWORD

I believe world peace is possible, and believe it starts with each and every one having total well-being – mind, body, spirit. At the time I write this book, mental health is of growing concern in our society. Every year, as many as 20-25% of all Americans experience some type of mental illness, such as depression, which arguably is ranked as the second leading cause of disability in the U.S, as well as around the world.[123]

My intent is that *Vibrant Happy You* guides you towards your own personal, total well-being. I hope in the pages of this book you find simple practices that will make a lasting and profound difference in your mental, physical and spiritual well-being, so that you can be and experience your true self, contributing your gifts and talents to the world.

In my opinion, an amazing life is the reason we come to earth. <u>You have a purpose</u>. You have so much to offer the world, you matter, and most importantly, you CAN be peaceful and happy. To me, our destiny and purpose on this earth is to have fun and enjoy life to the fullest extent possible. I truly believe that if you are not having fun, you're doing it wrong.

I am excited to share my story and all I have learned throughout my personal wellness journey, that it might serve to provide you relief and be a catalyst for a quantum leap in your path towards being the best you and living your best life. ~ Namaste

CHAPTER 1:
GETTING STARTED

Congratulations! The fact that you are reading this book means that you or someone you love has the awareness to recognize and acknowledge that there are times in life that you get sad, depressed, anxious and/or stressed. If you do not recognize or acknowledge that you are experiencing these emotional states, there is nothing you can do to address them. If you did not believe there is a solution or a better way, you would not be reading these words. Awareness is the first step, and the beginning of any journey is the toughest. I honor and acknowledge you for picking up this book and taking an action that will positively impact your life and change the course of your depression and/or anxiety story. I acknowledge you for your commitment to your health and well-being. Thank you for loving yourself. **You are worth it**.

This book is a guide to support you in designing your own personal road map for your optimal well-being journey. To help create your story, it is best to read the chapters in sequential order the first time through. This is because each habit or practice described in the following pages builds on the preceding practice. You will reap the benefits of each practice through repetition, implementation, and application as they begin to evolve into habits that require less energy and effort.

The approach laid out here is holistic. All the practices are inter-connected and include the mind, body, and spirit (or soul). All three realms are connected. It is only by addressing all of them that you can re-establish balance, to address the stress and false beliefs that you have when you are feeling depressed, anxious, or both. These seven practices are now habits for me and have helped me transform my mental, physical and emotional well-being. You too can practice and implement each on a regular basis in your life in a way that works for you until they become your healthy habits. If you take on the practices outlined in this book, you can discover the many layers of you and your well-being that impact your mental and emotional health.

After applying the practices in order, you can apply them as you choose in future use. For now, I recommend setting aside time to implement them daily. A workbook is provided at the end of the book to guide you step-by-step in putting the practices into action so that you can develop them into healthy habits to live your best life. I recommend you have a journal with you while reading this, so you can take notes, reflect, and have additional writing space if needed when completing the workbook exercises.

With the help of an amazing artist, Ilana Cloud, I have also included beautiful mandalas with affirmations, quotes and reminders at the end of this book for you to cut out or post up somewhere you will see them.

I know, firsthand, that amazing mental and emotional well-being is possible for anyone suffering from depression or anxiety. Love yourself and trust yourself and the universe enough to put these simple practices into action for at least 21 days and then beyond to transform your life, one day at a time.

You are worth it, and everyone whose life you touch is waiting for you to be your best you.

COMMITMENT TO YOURSELF

This journey can be very rewarding and transform your life in positive ways. To get the full benefit, it will take your commitment and willingness to do the work required. In addition to setting aside time, doing the exercises, and taking action, it will involve a mental, physical and spiritual shift to welcome and connect to your inner wisdom, peace and joy. To start you on the path to realizing your inner joy, make a commitment to yourself for at least 21 days and allow yourself to discover new ways of being and living. *Choose to be wholeheartedly committed, even when times get tough or other priorities creep in.* Mindfully, resist reverting to old, familiar ways.

I once heard that to fully experience being alive, one must step out onto the skinny branches, take risks and be courageous. It is easy to say and easy to dream of, and not always so easy to be, do, and live that way if we don't truly believe it's possible. To live the healthy, happy life we truly desire, we must reprogram our mind and believe with mind, body and soul that the life we desire is absolutely possible and out there waiting for us to connect to it.

The moment I made a commitment to myself to be 100% responsible for my life and to put my happiness above all else was the moment my life changed. I have learned to no longer let anything bother me for more than a few minutes, if that. I can say with 100% certainty that I am happy every day.

I want you to get the most out of the tools in this book; therefore, *I ask that you agree to commit to giving yourself 100% to creating your health and happiness story.* The commitment or pledge to yourself as written on the next page is a guide, so feel free to amend as you see fit, and once you do, sign it. Sign right in the book or rewrite your commitment and sign in your journal.

My Commitment to Myself

I_____, understand that I am undertaking an amazing 21-day journey. I commit wholeheartedly to creating lifelong health and happiness for myself. I commit to keeping a journal and completing all the exercises in the pages and workbook. I make my peace, joy and happiness a priority from this day forward. I love and accept myself deeply and completely. I commit to taking this journey ONE day at a time and promise to be loving, kind and generous with myself from this day forward.

_____   _____

Signature   Date

CHAPTER 2:
MY STORY

Now that you understand how to use the tools in this book, let me share with you how I got to this stage in my journey.

Growing up, I heard a lot of stories about mental illness being part of my genes. My father talked about how his dad committed suicide on the train tracks in the little town of Murillo, Spain where he was born. Then, many years later, his brother, my uncle, committed suicide on the same train tracks. I heard depression was common and that it was an illness that ran in the family. I remember as a young child feeling very lonely and isolated, sad that I had no family other than my parents and my sisters in the U.S. Holidays, birthdays and special occasions were events with my parents, sisters and family friends that we called uncle, aunts and cousins. But I remember always thinking, where is my "real family?" I remember feeling different and not understood — the only ½ Ecuadorian ½ Spanish girl at my school (other than my sisters). I did not feel like I belonged, and all these thoughts and beliefs contributed to the deep sadness I felt and endless nights crying myself to sleep, wondering why my parents had left their countries to be here in the U.S. all alone. I did not have many friends. I felt that I couldn't really relate or connect with people. I felt separate and different, and therefore, kept my distance, feeling much more comfortable keeping to myself. My story of being alone very much influenced my desire to go as far away to college as possible, where I truly would know no one. Ironically, I chose a college with less than a 5% Hispanic population, so if I felt different in the very diverse high school in northern New Jersey, I felt like an alien at the all-white college in New England.

Right before going away to college and several thoughts of what ending my life might be like, I saw my first therapist. While attending college, I began seeing a therapist weekly, who soon recommended I see a psychiatrist to prescribe medications. Medications that were supposed to take away the chemical imbalance that caused the low moods, loneliness, deep sadness and feelings of isolation, stress and anxiety I experienced on a daily basis.

At that time in my life, I was an overachiever and perfectionist, and I put a lot of pressure on myself and others. I worked hard and worried a lot. I felt I had to study harder, longer, take more detailed notes, do extra credit, go above and beyond. This self-destructive cycle would exhaust me mentally, physically and emotionally, causing me to sometimes be anxious or depressed, and sometimes both. I would worry about the future and be depressed about what I did not have, did not know how to get; all these missing things I thought I "should" have or "should" be. The worst part is, I had no awareness of how I was. I was just being myself. I did not know how not to worry, and even more frightening, I didn't even know I was worrying. I simply thought I was being proactive, being prepared, ensuring I thought through worst case scenarios in order to have success. I believed worrying was necessary in order to plan, prepare and anticipate to make sure things turned out well. Other people who didn't worry were not me; they didn't need to worry whether things came easier for them or if they had support systems, family and friends. I didn't have an easy life, so I had to do it myself.

This mindset and way of being manifested itself in physical health issues. I would often get stomach upsets, have poor digestion, get headaches and chest pains. I remember for years having an upset stomach before school each day and vomiting nothing every morning, being nervous about going to school. My chest pains increased, and after seeing a few doctors to determine the cause, one doctor said I had a heart murmur.

Over the years, I saw several therapists and psychiatrists and tried several medications for depression and anxiety. Nothing I tried made a difference; I never seemed to feel better. I never left a session with my therapist or psychiatrist empowered or that I was ok. Despite several different antidepressants and regular adjustments to my dosages, I never felt like I was making progress.

One summer, when I was home from college, I couldn't remember the new dosage change in my meds, and I took too many and ended up in the hospital. I don't remember the experience much at all; in fact, I don't remember much about that time in my life. Memories are blurry; I was low energy and low mood much of the time. The start of my wake-up call for a better solution came when one increase in my antidepressant sent me on a manic episode, and I almost lost my job. I immediately switched psychiatrists as I no longer trusted that one. I switched doctors and was labeled bipolar and put on another medication to stabilize me and balance my moods. It was after being on my bipolar meds of about a year that I noticed I no longer felt anything. The bipolar meds were supposed to stabilize me so that I wouldn't experience extreme lows. However, I didn't experience highs either. My happy feelings were gone. I didn't feel like me anymore. I didn't know who I was. There was no joy, and when I realized this, I told my psychiatrist I no longer wanted to continue on medications, and she worked with me to lower my dosage slowly and taper off.

I knew there was a better way. I didn't know what or how, but part of me knew. I had faith that there was something better out there for me, and my journey led me to lots of teachers, mentors and experts, and I began to move into the awareness of my own power. I began practicing yoga regularly. I completed a transcendental meditation training and began meditating daily. I attended courses and completed several programs designed to empower me and reprogram my brain from limiting beliefs to empowered beliefs. I continued reading books on success, manifesting my desires, wealth, and anything that piqued my interest in the area of growth, development and abundant living.

In 2011, after practicing many of the tools and techniques shared here for about a year, I rewrote my story of not being athletic and created myself as an athlete, trained and completed my first of five half-marathons. Soon after, I did a diet program that taught about weight loss, energy sources, and the human body. I was so successful losing 25 lbs. of fat and building five pounds of muscle mass in three months that I began coaching others on the protocol. After years of wellness coaching, in 2015, I became a 200-Hour Registered Yoga Instructor and started Ananda Total Wellbeing, a holistic wellness practice empowering women to love the way they look and feel. I combined my master's degree and experience in Organizational Psychology, wellness and life coaching, essential oils, yoga and fitness instruction to empower clients to achieve results.

I hope that my journey and my relentless drive to having a vibrant, healthy life will serve as inspiration, as well as a resource for you to find your path and your journey to the best you.

We are all unique, AND we are all human beings. As such, we have more commonalities than differences. This holistic approach takes into account all aspects of human nature to guide you back to your natural state of well-being, back to balance and provide you with the practices you can regularly implement to create healthy habits for life — habits that will bring balance to your mind, body and spirit.

CHAPTER 3:
AWARENESS OF MIND

Let's start your journey by looking at the role your mind plays in shaping your wellness. Your choices are influenced by your thoughts and beliefs, which both consciously and unconsciously shape your life. However, for many of us, most of our thoughts and beliefs are unconscious. We are not aware of them, yet they affect every area of our lives and have enormous impacts on our feelings, actions and inactions.

The choices you make each day contribute to your health and well-being. Many of the choices you make have become unconscious habits; some serve you while others do not. Until the unconscious is made conscious, you have little power or knowledge to make the changes or shifts in your life that would serve you in being the best version of yourself. Once you uncover the unconscious beliefs and habits that have been in the way, you can more easily discover your peace, joy and happiness. You can author your new story and take control of your life.

Beliefs are views that you have thought repeatedly over a period of time. Webster's dictionary defines beliefs as, *"something one accepts as true or real; a firmly held opinion or conviction."* Your recurrent thoughts are beliefs you hold so firmly that they become your story and influence the way you see the world. They create your point of view and interpretation of a person, subject, situation, or circumstance — about everything. Consider this; events and circumstances are neutral, alone they have no meaning. It is the interpretation and meaning you place on each that influences your thoughts, emotions and behaviors.

Your brain is designed to process information through your thoughts. An influential mentor and teacher, T. Harv Eker, to whom I am very grateful, says, *"your inner world creates your outer world."* If your brain produces thoughts of inner peace and joy, you will find yourself experiencing a peaceful and joyful life.

Your interpretation of the world is part of your survival mechanism, and it exists for you to make sense of everything around you. To understand your environment, you subconsciously judge, assess, and assign meaning to everything in your environment so that you can make moment-to-moment decisions. This thinking and interpreting of data through our senses is what makes us as humans unique from other species. To become consciously aware of your thoughts, you want to recognize that these judgements and assessments you ascribe to your thoughts are not reality, but rather interpretations of reality based on your previous experiences, events and conditioning.

There is enormous freedom in the awareness of not believing each thought you have and knowing that each thought is not the truth. Unfortunately, these judgements, assessments and misperceptions are not pointed only at the world — we are our own worst enemy and critic. We judge, assess and criticize ourselves and our own actions constantly. I believe we as human beings have an innate desire to be better than we are today and to have the best that we can have, and somewhere along the way, we were erroneously taught, observed, and came to believe that by judging, assessing and trying to figure things out, we can accomplish our desire to be better.

I have come to learn the opposite is true. Judging, criticizing and being hard on yourself does not allow you the freedom to be, do, and have any of what you desire. Instead, it holds you back and limits you from being able to create, receive and take the necessary actions to accomplish your dreams.

We all experience what I call the *Cycle of Thoughts to Action*.

For example, the thoughts that I had as a child and young adult convinced me that I was alone, different, and that no one understood me. This created feelings of sadness, loneliness and frustration within me. My thoughts had me seeing myself as separate and isolated from people and made me believe that the world was an unloving place, and that life was hard. My attempts to interpret and make sense of my world as I saw it were in vain because I misperceived everything that was happening around me from that story and point of view.

Over time, I became very angry. I began to believe that life was unfair and that I did not belong. These beliefs contributed to more feelings of sadness, emptiness and hopelessness, which, in turn, affected my actions. I would cry myself to sleep every night and not share myself with my classmates, preferring instead to remain isolated and keep to myself. I did not see that these actions caused me to sink further into sadness and depression. When I would cry, my mind would race, and more negative thoughts would enter my head. I would begin to worry and ask myself questions such as, "Will I be alone forever?" "Will I ever have a friend that understands me?" "Will I ever fit in?" My mind would race on and on down this destructive thought pattern, causing my breathing to become more and more shallow. With each thought I would get sadder, my breath would get shallower, and I would literally curl my body into a small ball, reducing my ability to breathe deeply. This led me to hyperventilate and cry to the point of exhaustion. It was only then that I would finally fall asleep.

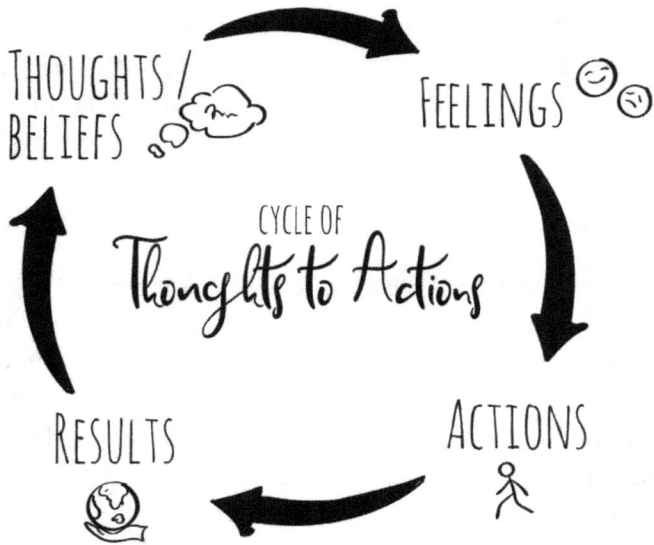

CYCLE OF
Thoughts to Actions

THOUGHTS / BELIEFS

FEELINGS

ACTIONS

RESULTS

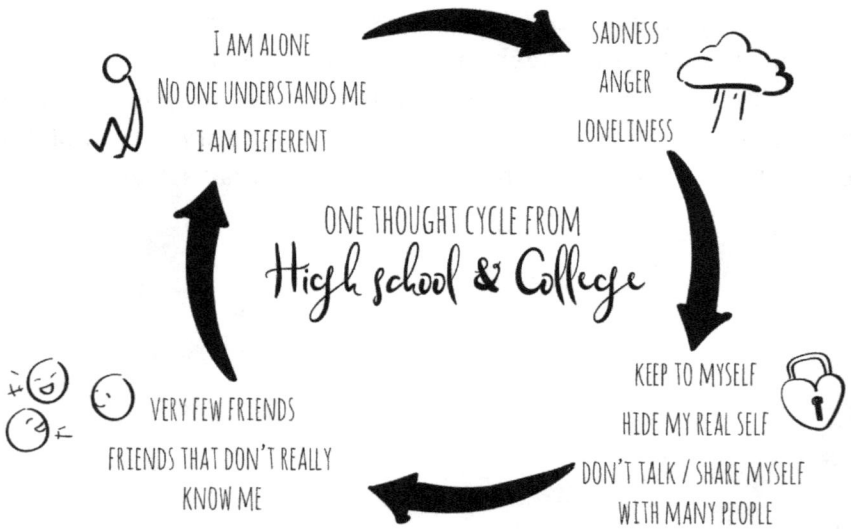

ONE THOUGHT CYCLE FROM
High school & College

I AM ALONE
No ONE UNDERSTANDS ME
I AM DIFFERENT

SADNESS
ANGER
LONELINESS

KEEP TO MYSELF
HIDE MY REAL SELF
DON'T TALK / SHARE MYSELF
WITH MANY PEOPLE

VERY FEW FRIENDS
FRIENDS THAT DON'T REALLY
KNOW ME

As my example shows, thoughts can have a huge impact on your life. Thoughts that drain your energy and hold you back from having what you want and desire are what I refer to as *limiting beliefs*. Limiting beliefs such as, "I can't," "it's too hard," "I shouldn't," that "it's not possible," and other false interpretations constrain you. If we consider that thoughts are like energy, we know from the scientific law of attraction that like attracts like.

A thought that has you feeling sad, upset, or produces any low energy emotion will automatically welcome or attract other similar thoughts. This will keep bringing you more of the same low energy feelings and emotions. This is why it is easy to spiral into low moods of sadness and depression or into thoughts of worry that have you anxious. The power of awareness means that by noticing this and catching your thoughts early in the process, you possess the key to turning around the downward spiral of thoughts and emotions that can lead to anxiety or depression. So, how can you do this? If you can take a deep breath, you can slow down your thoughts and create a pause; then you can consciously choose another thought that supports you in the moment. We'll explore the power and benefits of deep breathing more in Chapter 7 (page 35).

Remember, there is nothing wrong with you. There is nothing about you or others you need to fix or change. You are perfect just the way you are. By loving yourself and accepting yourself and your circumstances, you will find the space to shift them. Real change comes not from changing yourself, but rather from the awareness that there is nothing wrong, nothing to change.

Another personal example of how our unconscious thoughts can affect us comes from a time, many years ago, when I was barely speaking with my younger sister. I would pick up the phone to call her, and I would think to myself, *"I know she will hang up on me, or she never wants to talk to me, so I need to make this fast before she hangs up."* The conversation would go something like this: "Hi, listen, I need you to take mom to the doctor next week. Did you take care of the arrangements for the food next weekend, and what time will you be arriving at mom's?" I would rush to get through my questions, and my tone was harsh. There was no love or affection because my anxiety about her hanging up on me would take over the moment I picked up the phone.

It was not until I took a course, The Landmark Forum, that I realized it was my thoughts that led to my emotions and actions rather than reality, that kept me separate and disconnected from my sister. The fear of having her hang up on me or speak to me in a way I perceived as nasty kept me from sharing myself and my life with her. My thoughts kept me from building the relationship I wanted with my sister. What I noticed when I looked to see how I was being with her, rather than blaming her, I saw that my tone – demanding attitude – and the way I rushed to get what I needed, would have anyone hang up on me. I was downright unpleasant to talk to! It was this awareness of myself and my limiting beliefs in the relationship and communication that allowed me to see new actions that I could take, actions that matched my desire to have love and connection with my sister.

Through the awareness of my limiting beliefs, I learned to notice my thoughts as separate from me and as the fears they were, rather than clinging on to them as the truth. I could see they were not real; I had made those thoughts up. They were my interpretations and beliefs from many previous interactions with my sister. With this newfound awareness, I realized that my sister might not actually dislike me and, that maybe she even wanted the same thing, which was a great harmonious relationship and friendship. That maybe she *did* want to talk to me but couldn't if her interpretation of my behavior was that I was unbearable.

It would benefit us greatly to let go of our misconceived thoughts, no matter how real they may seem. If you stop reliving the past experiences that you have misinterpreted in your life and focus on what you want in the present moment, you will have tremendous power. To do this, you must be aware of your thoughts and notice if based in the past. The past is the past, and there is nothing you or anyone can do about it today. It likely served some kind of purpose in your life, and you can add negative meaning or positive meaning to the situation.

It is by becoming aware of your mind, body and soul's desires that you consciously create the life of joy, happiness and peace you desire every moment. Rather than being a victim of your circumstances and stories, through awareness, you can begin to consciously choose our thoughts. Aligning your thoughts with your desires brings harmony. For example, thinking that your sister, friend, co-worker, whoever you desire a relationship with may also want a relationship with you rather than they do not will allow you to experience peace or harmony, and in this space, you can take different actions to further what you want for that relationship.

CHAPTER 4:
PRACTICE 1: MEDITATION

Now that you are becoming more aware of your thoughts, let's look at the first practice to forward your journey. One powerful way to begin to bring awareness to the *Cycle of Thoughts to Actions* and your limiting beliefs is meditation. Meditation is the embodiment of awareness and is the first practice for your health and happiness. Meditation is often misunderstood. Many people think it's difficult or that they can't meditate because they can't clear their mind or make it blank. They are correct. Clearing your mind or making it blank is nearly impossible. It requires years of practice, and even then, it may not happen. This is not surprising since as mentioned in Chapter 2, the brain is designed to constantly assess and process information for our survival.

So what then is meditation? It is a practice of focusing and going inward and past the layers of the mind. Meditation is powerful because by going inward, being aware of, and witnessing your thoughts, you start to have access to your unconscious thoughts and beliefs. The mind and its constant activity will still be there, and you simply notice or become aware of your mind, your body, your breath, and simply be in the moment. During meditation, you are aware of everything, while at the same time bringing your focus to one thing. Depending on your method of meditation, the focal point can be your breath, a mantra, or a candle flame. By bringing your attention and awareness back to the single focal point, you slowly learn to tame the mind, to slow it down, to quiet the thought-chatter. In meditation, you accept all that is, just as it is, you notice your thoughts and let them go, free of judgement or attachment. You let each thought that arises float away, each body sensation pass and keep bringing back your attention and awareness to your mantra, your breath or your chosen focal point. You begin by connecting with your breath to tune inward. As you practice meditation and relax more into your body, focus on your breathing and be gentle with your thoughts, you will begin to increase the space between your thoughts, and in that gap of silence, experience peace.

During meditation, as the observer or witness of your thoughts, you gain greater awareness of yourself. You realize that you have thoughts, but that they are not you. Over time, the practice of awareness will allow you to be more present when you are not meditating as well. With regular and consistent practice, you can experience the numerous benefits of meditation, such as the ability to quiet the mind for longer and longer periods, greater clarity and self-awareness, peace, tranquility, and the ability to respond rather than react.

Meditation is a powerful tool. It can support you in being more focused, aware, mindful and productive throughout your day. According to the National Center for Complementary and Integrative Health at the National Institutes of Health (NIH), meditation has a long history of use in increasing calmness and physical relaxation, improving psychological balance, coping with illness and enhancing overall health and well-being.[5]

Meditation can have a transformative impact on your life, and with time, quiet your mind to reduce anxiety and stress. When you meditate, you become aware of your emotions, which increases your self-awareness and perspective. This, in turn, provides you with clarity to perform and be at your best.

The practice of meditation can look like you sitting quietly for 10-15 minutes, and during this time, your body and mind are given this precious time to be still, relax and just be. As you focus internally on your breath and get present in the moment, fully relaxed, you will begin to connect to your true self and discover your inner peace. In the quiet space between the thoughts that will inevitably arise, you will find silence within and experience peace. In that silence, you will also experience joy: nothing to do, nothing to prove, nothing to get right. As you cease judging your thoughts and simply let them float away as easily as they floated in, you will experience separation from your thoughts and the awareness that you are not your thoughts, and even though you have them, these thoughts are separate from you. Thoughts do not define you. They are simply impulses of energy, and you can let them go, judgement-free — nothing good, nothing bad, just thoughts. In this awareness that you have, you are not your thoughts, you can experience the freedom to simply be. Yogis say the entire universe is within, because in the silence in-between your thoughts, you can experience peace, joy, love and freedom. With consistent practice, the silent space in between the thoughts grows longer. In time, you can create greater peace, joy, love, and freedom for yourself and your life, during, as well as after meditation.

Meditation can be a great tool for training the mind not to be distracted and caught up in endless thoughts that do not serve or empower you. Meditation teaches you to take notice and to be present and aware of what is taking place around you so that you can respond, rather than react to what you experience. It brings you freedom from the mind and its meandering, and, in this freedom, you experience who you truly are; distinct from your mental turmoil. This is where you find inner peace. As you apply the principle of meditation to your life, you can be fully aware of what is going on. Continual practice of meditation can be a means of freeing yourself from worries and allow you the freedom to experience the joy of being fully present in the here and now, which is all we have.

After a couple of years of meditating daily, one of the unexpected benefits that I began experiencing is effortlessly discovering solutions to my problems. A clear example was a few years ago, after implementing many of these tools in my life, when I was preparing to move to California. I was planning my going away party, and my one-bedroom condo was not large enough to fit all the friends I wanted to invite. My criteria were simple: I wanted a place with a fun ambiance that I didn't need to pay for that could accommodate at least 30 people, so I could have a wonderful send-off surrounded by all my friends. I wracked my brain for weeks but could not come up with one that met all my requirements. One day while meditating, a thought that arose was Los Tios Restaurant. The thought of the restaurant and its back room floated into my mind; problem solved. I let the thought go and continued meditating. After meditating, I called the restaurant and made a reservation in the back room. I created a Facebook invite and invited all my friends to my going away party at Los Tios Restaurant, which met all my criteria; we met there for the party, and everyone had a fabulous time.

I know of others who meditate and find solutions by asking direct questions. I have had some success with this, and others I know can ask a question to their higher self at the beginning of their meditation and listen and receive an answer during meditation. It's truly amazing how much clarity, understanding and wisdom can come during these silent moments. When you get quiet and let go of trying to figure things out, force an outcome, get it right or perfect, you can listen to your inner wisdom that has the best answers. Usually, in the course of our daily living, we simply do not get quiet enough to hear them.

Through the practice of meditation, you can begin a practice of noticing your thoughts, feelings and body sensations as you move through life during and after meditation. When you experience a stressful event or moment, be aware of what you are thinking and feeling physically and emotionally. With this awareness, you can slow down your racing, protective, caveperson brain, bring separation and space to you and your thoughts, and then choose who you want to be and what you want to do at that moment. If this doesn't happen at first, it's ok. Keep practicing! Having self-awareness allows you to see where your thoughts and emotions are taking you. When you have awareness, you can choose something different — a different thought, emotion or action. In this heightened state of awareness, you can immediately make better choices in your thought processes and your emotional reactions. The key is catching and noticing your behaviors early in the process *before* you act.

"Meditation is an adventure, an exploration, and sometimes a discovery of a land inside we did not know existed."[6] I trained at "Mind the Mat Yoga & Pilates," and they have a great analogy and teaching on meditation that likens the phases of meditation we pass through to a three-phase weather system.

The first phase, Dharana, involves the use of concentration techniques. When you first begin meditating, there is a lot going on in your head. It is as if you are in a fog. It is helpful to have a focal point like a flashlight to guide you and ground you as you move forward slowly through the fog that is the process of meditation. The second phase is Dhyana, which is a state of willfulness and surrender. In this phase, you begin to enter the "flow," and the fog begins to lift. Your vision expands, and your meditation begins to feel more natural and less forced. The third phase is Samadhi, which is full surrender and presence in the moment. In this phase, you surrender completely to all that is and are in a state of pure being, and your experience is like that of sunny, clear weather. However, the process is not linear. There may be times during your meditation that you go back and forth from flow to fog with brief moments of sun. The true practice of meditation is not to arrive anywhere, but rather to instill and experience a deep acceptance of yourself in each moment.

There are various ways to meditate, and there is a meditation technique that will work for you. Experimenting to discover what works for you can be fun. We are all dynamic beings, ever-changing and evolving, so the type of meditation you practice over time may change. The joy is in trying out and practicing different types of meditations to see which one works for you today.

In the workbook at the end of this book, you will find guided meditations and instructions for you to begin or expand your meditation practice. You can also visit my website, www.clarav.com for video and audio guided meditations and more.

TIP:

Try out a meditation App, such as:

- The Mindfulness App

- Headspace

- Calm

- Insight Timer

CHAPTER 5:
PRACTICE 2: DECLARATION

As we have seen, meditation can bring you to a place of clarity and calmness, allowing you to reprogram and create new empowering beliefs to influence your emotions and actions. Now, let's explore the second practice, declaration, in which you speak out loud into existence your desires in order to create what you want in the world. Creating and speaking thoughts and beliefs that empower you toward your goals and desires begins the process of reprogramming your brain for success. Through repetition, thinking and speaking new thoughts, you can rewire your brain to create new neural pathways of new thoughts, beliefs and emotions that allow for a life full of joy and happiness.

You can create a new *Thought to Action Cycle*. Think about how you want to feel, who you want to be, and begin speaking and sharing that. Begin authoring your life and rewriting your story by speaking your desires and bringing them to life. Remember to go easy on yourself, it took many years to engrain your limiting beliefs into your subconscious, so it will take time, patience and consistent awareness to consciously create your new empowering beliefs through declaration. Declaration is an intentional process, you are not speaking wishes or wants but rather making explicit statements or pronouncements out loud. Announce to yourself and the world, your friends, the people in your life who you are and how you feel purposely and see how things start to shift. Speak your intentions and desires positively for yourself and others to hear.

By repeatedly declaring and speaking positive affirmations and adding feeling as you involve your entire body, you can reprogram old ways of thinking, being and acting. Stand tall or sit up tall, have your chest be open and speak out loud what it is you are declaring for yourself and your future. Saying the new thoughts regularly out loud will help to reshape your thinking and over time turn into new automatic thoughts that are more positive and aligned to who you want to be, moment by moment. As you begin to transition your thoughts, begin to make positive meaning out of the experiences and situations in your life. When things don't work or go the way you want, when your intention is not realized, or your expectation is not met, think and say something positive about it, anyway. There is always something positive you can find about any situation, circumstance or event; ALWAYS. Keeping a positive mindset about any situation will allow you to think more clearly and act wisely in the moment.

When you become aware of a thought that produces negative energy, or a thought that starts a thought to action cycle scenario you do not want to continue, become your own best friend by talking back lovingly to yourself. Be a voice of kindness, acceptance, and forgiveness. Separate yourself from your thoughts and notice they are not true, they are simply energetic impulses that come and go. When you notice a thought that has you feeling low or any undesirable feeling for you, replace it with a thought that has you feeling better, good, or more positive. What thought would most serve you now to bring you peace, calmness and joy in that moment? By noticing your thoughts and words, you can consciously and purposefully replace old thoughts and speaking that does not support your true intention. When you notice a limiting belief, say "thank you for sharing, AND I believe..." and create something wonderful. When you notice you've said something limiting, catch yourself and don't finish saying it or say something positive immediately after, "what I really meant to say was..."

The thought, choice, and declaration I made in 2010 to be 100% committed to my happiness above all else made a huge difference in my life from that day forward. It allowed me to say to myself during difficult times that I may not like this right now, but no matter what, I am going to be happy, and I will get through this. This new thought process and moment-by-moment way of thinking allowed me to create a new belief that I can be happy, no matter what, because I chose to be, because I said so. Rather than staying upset, frustrated or disappointed because I had those feelings, thoughts and body sensations that came along with them, I said to myself, *I'm going to be happy, no matter what, and will not let this bother me one more second*. Sometimes I would say it in my head, sometimes I would say it to whomever I was with. I would say things like, "OK, I am not going to get upset" or "I'm going to make the best of this," or "OK, all I can do is laugh." It was a whole new way of living for me. From the commitment and promise I made to myself and declaring it out loud, I began thinking, speaking and being happier each day.

It's amazing how when you speak your desires and intentions out loud in the world people and events begin showing up to support you. Ralph Waldo Emerson said, "Once you make a decision, the universe conspires to make it happen." I would continue this by saying that after making the decision AND declaring it out loud for others to hear is how people around you can support you in having that.

CHAPTER 6:
AWARENESS OF BODY

We saw in Chapter Three that there is great freedom and power in being mentally self-aware. Now, let us transition out of the mind, and move into another realm – the body. Awareness of your body is a powerful tool for your health and well-being. Connecting and tuning into your body moves you out of your thoughts and the worrying mind so that you can be present in the moment, rather than regretting the past or worrying about the future. When you tune in and listen to your body, it has an amazing way of healing and bringing itself back into balance.

What happens in your body, for example, your posture and the way you carry yourself, also influences your mind and mood. Embodied cognition is the philosophy based on the idea that the relationship between your mind and body runs both ways, that your mind influences your body and that your body posture also affects your mind.[7] Think about how you carry yourself when you are sad or feel down. I know I used to curl myself into a ball, wrap myself up tight in a blanket on the couch, sit hunched over in front of my computer, or slouch wherever I was sitting. In each of these postures, I was literally making myself smaller, contracting my body and rounding my neck and shoulders forward with my head down. Think about how you hold your body when you feel happy, alive, excited. When I am happy, present and engaged, I'm sitting up tall or standing up tall, I'm making eye contact with whatever or whomever I'm attentive to. When I need to present in front of an audience, I stand tall with a little puff in my chest to be and look confident. In a series of experiments, researchers found that sitting in a collapsed, helpless position makes it easier for negative thoughts and memories to appear, while sitting in an upright, powerful position makes it easier to have empowering thoughts and memories. "Emotions and thoughts affect our posture and energy levels; conversely, posture and energy affect our emotions and thoughts," says one of Peper's studies from 2012.[8]

Similar to posture, the simple act of smiling can affect your mood as well as increase your happiness and decrease your stress. Smiling activates the release of neuropeptides that work toward fighting off stress. The feel-good neurotransmitters – dopamine, endorphins, and serotonin – are all released when a smile flashes across your face as well. This not only relaxes your body, but it can also lower your heart rate and blood pressure. The serotonin release brought on by your smile serves as an antidepressant or mood lifter. [9]

Having a greater awareness of your body and your posture allows you the opportunity to physically influence how you feel. Next time you are feeling down, notice your body posture, and in that moment, adjust your body, stand up or sit up, relax your shoulders, pull your shoulders back slightly to open your chest and sit or stand "confidently." Put on a smile, whether you feel like it or not and let the smile create your happier mood. Let your body support how you want to feel, and let your mind follow.

CHAPTER 7:
PRACTICE 3: DEEP BREATHING

Now that we have seen the power of awareness of both mind and body, let's explore practice three, which is deep breathing, and see how it works as a tool to facilitate your well-being. Breath is the connection between mind, body and spirit. Breath is life; it is the first thing we do when we are born and the last thing when our spirit departs our body. There is a circular interconnection between our thoughts, our mind, and our breathing because each is influenced by the other.[10]

The benefits of practicing deep breathing on a regular basis include reduced anxiety and depression as well as decreased feelings of stress or being overwhelmed. When you have thoughts that you perceive as negative or stressful, your sympathetic nervous system, which is responsible for your fight and flight responses, shifts from its normal maintenance level to high gear. It automatically regulates your breathing to become shallow and fast. You experience a sensation of shortness of breath since you are breathing only from the chest rather than from your diaphragm. You have no control over this instantaneous flight or fight survival response that we humans have had since the beginning of humanity. Your body immediately goes into high gear as soon as the stress message from the brain is sent. This automatic stress response is reversible the instant you create a sense of calm in your mind and body by breathing deeply and slowly.[10] Breathing deeply allows your heart rate to slow and return to normal, and as a result, produces a calming effect on the mind and body. Deep breathing also helps in calming and slowing any emotional turbulence in your mind. [11]

Deep breathing is a powerful tool to support you in influencing and managing how you want to think and feel, and proper use of your breath can empower you. For example, by practicing yoga on a regular basis, I learned to be mindful of my breathing, body and posture. Before yoga, I used to breathe very shallowly. Each time I would inhale, my shoulders would rise, demonstrating that I was breathing from my chest rather than my diaphragm. My overall posture did not support my well-being as I literally tended to try and protect my heart by rounding my back and bringing my shoulders forward towards one another. This posture closes off your ability to take in a full breath because it constricts your lung capacity. Sitting or standing tall with your chest slightly out and open, shoulder blades towards one another on your back, allows you to take full breaths. This is the same confident posture research discussed in chapter six that can influence feelings of confidence. Having your body assume a posture that facilitates deep, full breaths will allow your body and mind to be calmer.

Breathing effectively and efficiently is a vital and integral part of your journey to total well-being and helps with all the practices shared here. I have found deep breathing especially powerful for relieving my anxiety. Anxiety is usually accompanied by shallow breathing.[12] Therefore, slowing down your breathing and increasing your oxygen by breathing deeply can reverse the anxious state of both mind and body. I believe that similar to adjusting your posture to influence your feelings, adjusting your breathing in your body influences your mind and mood.

I remember it was in a yoga class that I learned how to breathe correctly. It's been life-changing and very calming to breathe deeply, the way we are designed to breathe. Notice babies' breathing; their belly will expand and fill up on the inhale and relax and their little shoulders relax on the exhale naturally. A baby doesn't learn to breathe this way, he or she does so instinctively, naturally, deeply from their tiny diaphragms.

It was during yoga class that I became aware that I was breathing exactly in the opposite way. The shallow way I was breathing was facilitating anxious feelings in my mind and body. When I would inhale, my belly would go in and my shoulders would rise. I actually was not filling my lungs with much air at all, and on the exhale, my belly would puff out and I would not release much air. This shallow chest breathing lent itself to regular panic attacks and a more anxious mind and body.

I remember after a few years of practicing yoga, and during my yoga teacher certification program, the power of bringing my awareness to and shifting my breathing. It was 3 A.M., I was sleeping next to my boyfriend at the time and his phone started getting all these texts. He was a heavy sleeper and didn't notice. I was a light sleeper and the texts disturbed my sleep. I reached over him for the phone on the nightstand to see who might be texting him at that hour. I looked at the phone and read the text, and to my shock, it was from another woman saying what a great time she had with him. I felt a sudden pressure in the middle of my chest and ran with the phone to the restroom. I wanted to read the entire chain of texts and figure out what was going on. I found a text from him telling her how much he had enjoyed spending time with her. A flood of emotion ran through my body. I was hurt, mad, angry. I felt so betrayed. I ran to the kitchen to get some air. I needed more space, more air; the tiny bathroom was too small. I was panicking, what do I do, how could this be happening to me? I thought we had such a good thing; I thought he was the one.

My breathing was now so shallow I was hyperventilating. At that moment, at the peak of my panic attack, a thought flashed into my head; calm down, take a deep breath. I turned to my yoga training, I brought my awareness to my breath and put my hand to my belly and took a deep breath, filling my diaphragm, ribs, then chest completely with air. I relaxed on the exhale, dropping my shoulders away from my ears, exhaling the air out my chest, ribs, then diaphragm. I took several long, deep breaths, and in seconds, my thoughts stopped swirling. I was now focused and in my body, and I could think clearly. I had a thought: "it's not the end of the world." I was not going to die as my hyperventilation had literally made me believe a few minutes earlier. I was calm, and I knew all there was to do was to have a conversation with him and get clear on what was really going on.

Through the practice of deep breathing, you can let go of all that does not serve you. You can use deep breathing to release stress, worry, icky feelings, and relax. You can use deep breathing to ease into your body or drop into your body and out of your head. As you inhale deeply, you can inhale clarity and peace. As you exhale, you can sink into your body, connect and ground, and experience a greater sense of peace and joy in the moment.

TIPS:

Be sure to be mindful of your breathing when you do the exercises in the workbook. Being mindful of your breathing and your posture will support you as you move through the practices, and in time, your habit will be to naturally breathe deeply.

Try out Breathe Apps like:

- The Breathe App

- Breathe In Calm App

CHAPTER 8:
PRACTICE 4: MOVEMENT

For your mind to be well, your body must also be well. The fourth practice is movement, and we will explore how all different kinds of movement can support you in living a vibrant, happy life. Many studies have shown that people who exercise regularly have lower rates of depression than those who do not.[13]

In our current day and age, we tend to be very sedentary. We sit all day in chairs, at our desks, in the car, on the couch, etc. During the many years I suffered from greater levels of depression and anxiety, I did not engage in regular physical activity. I did not work out, go to the gym, participate in any sports, get outdoors much, dance or move my body beyond walking to and from places. Physical activity and exercise were not something I was taught to value and prioritize, and as a young adult, I had a story or a set of beliefs that it was not enjoyable. My point of view was that it was work. When I reprogramed these old beliefs, which had contributed to my being overweight and moving very little, and began intentionally scheduling time for movement, exercise and getting outdoors, I felt good, positive, energized, alive, and accomplished. I created a new story, that with each activity, I had accomplished something positive for my health and body. I had gotten my butt out the door and done something good for my body when I wanted to stay on the couch. The best part: I felt really proud of myself.

Movement is a very clear way to feel into your body, connect with your body, and move out of your mind. It directly brings your attention to your body. It allows you the opportunity to focus your attention on the movement, the activity, the present moment in a very precise way. For example, when you are on a treadmill, your mind can wander and worry, but if it does and your pace starts to slow down or you mis-step, immediately, your body will let you know, and you'll be alerted back to pick up the pace, adjust the pace, or watch your footing. Same if you are biking or running; when your mind starts to wander too far off, the biker flying by you will remind you to come back to the bike and the road, or the squirrel crossing your path will bring you back to what you are doing in the present moment. In all physical activities, your body will bring your attention to your breath in order to keep on going. In all movement, your body will keep bringing you back out of your thoughts to your body and allow you the opportunity and reminder to notice your body and experience what it feels and what it is doing in the moment.

Physical exercise or sports activities also play an important part in our mental health because they help to dissipate emotional energy and release it harmlessly. In addition to releasing toxins from the body through sweat and increased circulation, blood flow and oxygen, exercise can help release emotions naturally.

Frustration, anger, upset, sadness, loneliness or any of our range of emotions are able to move through us when we engage in physical activities. I personally have experienced numerous runs where I let out my frustration, anger and upset on the pavement with each step I took or with each exhale. I can also remember several runs where I was sad and let my tears out as I ran (sweat or tears, no one needed to know the difference). I was able to do so because no one was on the road or path, and I was alone, comfortable enough for me to let out my emotions. By the end of the run, I had released some emotions and I felt good. I also know from doing yoga that moving into different postures in a flow yoga class has also allowed me to release feelings of sadness. During power yoga where I am sweating as I move, I have been able to release frustration from my day or week and leave feeling much more peaceful or energized – – depending on the sequence or routine.

Physical activity also supports your mental and emotional well-being because it triggers the release of endorphins, which make you feel good.[14] It is widely accepted that exercise reduces stress. After exercise, endorphins can help to lower heart rate and blood pressure, stabilize breathing and restore normal body temperature. Endorphin activity can also produce mild sedation, which may increase feelings of well-being and perceived relaxation after a workout. Other techniques, such as yoga, controlled-breathing exercises, and meditation, can also enhance the calming effects of endorphins after physical activity.[15]

Below are some movement suggestions and their benefits that I recommend. There may be some activities you know you enjoy doing that you simply do not make time to engage in regularly. As part of your commitment to yourself in this new phase of your journey, make the time, schedule the time, and make it happen. For your mental, physical and emotional well-being, it is vital that you enjoy and engage in daily movement. Some days, you may be able to fit in more movement than others. Use the Workbook at the end of this book (page 59) to put together a plan of how you will move daily and what days you can set aside longer periods for movement or exercise. Setting aside time to move, even in just 15-min intervals a few times a week, will make a difference.

Any movement or activity can range from gentle to intense. See how you can vary your movement routine to include a balance of both, depending on your fitness level and abilities. Always consult your doctor if you have any questions or concerns before beginning a new fitness routine.

Part of the 21-day plan is for you to choose a movement routine that works for you and begin incorporating movement regularly into your daily routine. Try starting with a minimum of 30 minutes of movement every day.

There are many gentle ways to begin incorporating movement into your daily activities. Walking can be a gentle way to move, especially if you are able to walk outside and connect with nature. Meditative walks can be wonderful as well because they allow you to practice mindfulness with each step. Meditative movement, or movement in which you pay attention to your bodily sensations, position in space, feelings, subtle changes in heart rate or breathing as you move, has been shown to alleviate depressive symptoms.[16] Qigong, Tai Chi and yoga are also helpful. Changing your posture, breathing and rhythm can all change your brain, thereby reducing stress, depression, and anxiety, and leading to a feeling of well-being.[17] To find out more, consider finding and attending some classes at your local YMCA, gym or fitness center, trying out a fitness app like Nike Training Club, 7 Minute Workout, or even using online videos as a guide on YouTube.

YOGA

Yoga is a practice that can range from gentle to intense and can be especially transformative. Yoga is meditation in movement. It can be practiced mindfully, bringing your awareness to your body and letting go of thoughts that arise that bring you away from your breath and body sensations and can teach non-judgement. You may hear the instructor say something like, "it's your practice, listen to your body," "it's not about getting it right, everyone's body is different," "do the best you can." In the Western world, there are many different kinds of yoga practices. My recommendation for those wanting to explore yoga for total mind-body health would be to try a few different classes at a local yoga studio or find some gentle or beginner yoga videos on YouTube, or search for a class in your area via the MindBody App.

There are a few easy yoga poses that I recommend to calm your mind and body and relieve stress provided in the Workbook Practice Four: Movement section that follows this book (page 70). These recommendations are simple enough to do daily, at home, on your own. A few minutes of deep breathing in the following yoga poses is a simple practice you can add to your day or week. To see video demonstrations, visit my website, www.clarav.com.

TIP:

Take 2 – 15 min breaks each day to walk outside, even in a parking lot, to get sunshine and fresh air

Practice declarations here too.

DANCE

Dance is another great way to get out of your head and into your body. As you dance, you move and release built up energy and emotions, thus improving mood and overall sense of well-being. Dance has the ability to bring you to a calm state of mind, as you focus on your body and your movements rather than your thoughts and worries. Studies on the effectiveness of dance movement therapy concluded that dancing should be encouraged as part of treatment for anxiety and depression.[18]

Partnered dancing can be especially great for some because of the added benefit of human contact. Having human contact in a way that is fun and aerobic, like dance, is a great way to relieve stress and anxiety and boost your mood. If you are able to surrender and let your partner lead, partnered dance can be an amazing experience to practice letting go; surrender, go with the flow, connect with another human being, and have fun. As the female partner in a dance, you must surrender and let the male partner lead. When you can do so and allow someone to guide you, as you feel and move with his communication and movements, you can experience the joy of simply being and allowing. Dancing with someone else is like exercise and a hug combined.

I know for a long time, for me and for many people today, that partnered dance or dance that requires steps and/or a partner is anxiety provoking rather than fun and relaxing. If that sounds true for you, I recommend taking some dance classes to build confidence and gain all the benefits mentioned above. You can search for a nearby Arthur Miller Dance Studio or MeetUp.com for dance lessons in your area. If you prefer to dance by yourself without a partner or any steps, search for Ecstatic Dance events near you.

MUSIC & MOVEMENT

However, no partner is needed to get the benefits of dancing. Putting on a song you enjoy that makes you want to move is all you need. Turn the music up and move freely, let your arms swing, let your feet and legs move as they wish. Jump, bob, spin, swirl, sway, move however you are called to move. Move however feels good and enjoy it. Dancing freely like there is no right or wrong way to dance (because there isn't) can be very liberating. You can make it a form of your expression, rather than something that you have to be good at or get right. Listen to uplifting music with a rhythm or beat that calls you to move. If you relax into dancing and let your body move with the music, it can also be meditative and stress-relieving. Focus on the movement; your body in space; your feet on the ground and breathe deeply. Enjoying the movement of your body in this way can center you and help you stay balanced. A healthy lifestyle is integrating the mind, body and soul relationship, and dance has all of those characteristics.

Music lifts mood, reduces anxiety, raises motivation and helps combat insomnia and depression. Soothing music can also have a calming therapeutic effect on our minds and bodies. Music has a unique link to our emotions, and can, therefore, be an effective stress management tool. A recent study by Stanford University shows that depressed patients gain self-esteem and their mood improves after music therapy.[19] Research from controlled treatment outcome studies has shown that listening to and playing music is a powerful treatment for mental health issues.[20] Music has positive physical effects as it can produce direct biological changes, such as reducing heart rate, blood pressure and cortisol levels.[21]

Music, similar to dance, can allow you to focus your attention on the sounds you hear, the vibrations you feel within physically and at the soul level, and allow you to tune into something greater and get you out of your head. For this reason, music can be a great aid to meditation, helping to prevent the mind wandering as easily.

Try dancing at home first if that feels better, and then get out there and dance!

TIP:

Use Pandora or Spotify playlists to get you going!

CHAPTER 9:
AWARENESS OF EMOTIONS AND SOUL

Moving deeper within, past the physical body to the realm of your spirit or soul, let's explore how awareness of your emotions play an integral part in your overall well-being. Emotions are natural and normal, and all humans have a range of emotions. Having an awareness of your emotions can allow you to move through difficulties faster by using your emotions as a navigation tool. Many of us do not allow ourselves to feel and experience the wide range of emotions we have as human beings. We falsely believe expressing certain emotions like anger, upset, sadness, disappointment or fear, to name a few, makes us weak, is bad, is negative, feels terrible, etc. We do not acknowledge these feelings, and we stuff them down, avoid them, or try to hide them. As mentioned above in the connection between our thoughts and feelings, it is important to allow your emotions and their energy move through you by movement, dance, and music through the physical body. This includes emotions you may not be as comfortable expressing. In writing this book, I discovered that depression is anger turned inwards. Anger unexpressed, unreleased and suppressed is detrimental to our well-being and living the life we love.

I recently experienced the impact of suppressing my sadness and unhappiness about my current living situation.

After months of ignoring my thoughts and feelings about it, and instead, telling myself it's not so bad, now is not the right time to focus on this, I'll think about this later, and distracting myself unconsciously to avoid dealing with this, I unknowingly became angry. I was on a call with someone, and she actually said to me, "Clara, why are you so angry?" Until that moment, I had no conscious idea or awareness of my anger.

Later that day and into the weekend, at a wellness retreat, the retreat leader said to me, "I notice you are not breathing deeply." I very quickly and curtly said, "Yes I am." She continued instructing me as the retreat was designed, and with each instruction, I grew more annoyed with her and angry. That's when it became really clear to me that I was, in fact, angry. I acknowledged my anger and frustration, and I expressed it saying to the course leader, "yes I am upset and annoyed at your instructions, I'm very frustrated." She suggested I release my anger through physical activity. I realized the anger had nothing to do with her; it had been building up. At the retreat, I had the space to release my anger through physical activity. I swung a bat, I punched a punching bag, and after some time doing that and having the anger, frustration and upset move through me, I stopped, took a deep breath, and started to cry. I realized underneath the anger I was really sad and unhappy to be living somewhere with such little social activities and opportunities for a single person. I got connected with my heart and my soul, and they both want to live somewhere beautiful and fun near the water.

I share this with you because I know from experience on this occasion, and many others, the freedom, peace and joy that comes from acknowledging whatever emotion I'm having, being with it and letting it pass, or being with it and discovering what I need to discover is perhaps underneath it in order to let it go. I also remember a time in the shower that I experienced a wave of sadness come over me, and at first, I resisted it and distracted myself by thinking about something else. I then remembered the importance of acknowledging my feelings. I had a thought, thanks to implementing all these practices, "just be with your feelings," so I allowed myself to experience the sadness, and in literally a minute, the sadness passed, and I actually laughed in the shower. I laughed because I had been afraid to feel sad, and there was nothing to be afraid of. I felt sad, and just as soon as it came, after experiencing it and being with it, it passed. Funny how what we are so afraid of isn't so scary after all.

I invite you to allow yourself to feel all your feelings. They can be expressed in constructive ways, explore and discover for yourself in speaking and physical activity what works for you. More intense exercise or movement and expressing with words what it is that you need to say are powerful tools for you to embrace and discover for yourself their magic.

TIPS:

Journal your feelings as well to express them and get them out onto paper.

Take a boxing, kickboxing class or self-defense class.

CHAPTER 10:
PRACTICE 5: REST & RELAXATION

To maintain balance, rest and relaxation are just as important as movement. Practice Five, rest and relaxation, allows you to take care of your whole being. Rest and relaxation are needed for the mind and body to operate at their best. Relaxation is the antidote for the tension and tightness caused by anxiety. A regular self-care routine and practice that includes several of the following relaxation components will allow you to experience greater balance and resilience in managing the stressors in your life. The benefits of deep relaxation include reduced general anxiety, reduced frequency and intensity of panic attacks, increased productivity and energy level, improved concentration and memory, reduced insomnia and fatigue, increased self-confidence and decreased overall stress levels.[22] A meta-analysis of several studies on relaxation training including meditation for anxiety show consistent and significant efficacy in reducing anxiety. [23]

The mind also has a role in your relaxation. An important part of relaxing is letting go, mentally and physically and accepting what is. Allow yourself to relax by letting go and forgiving yourself. Forgive yourself for all the things you've made yourself wrong about, for all the shoulds and expectations you have put on yourself. Let go of the need to control, the need to be perfect and get it right. It is this need for control and pressure we put on ourselves and others to be a certain way that leads to our anxiety and depression. Let the pressure you have been putting on yourself fall away.

Let it go and relax. Slow down; slow down your thoughts in order to be aware of them. Slow down your breathing to relax and calm your mind, body and emotions. Slowing down actions and the need to do do do and go go go. By slowing down, gaining awareness, clarity and inner wisdom, you will actually speed up and accelerate your success. You did not come to this earth to control everything and have it look a certain way. You came to live, to create, to dream big dreams and have those dreams come true. You are a human being. BE.

BE YOURSELF! BE FREE! BE EASY!

In addition to gentle or restorative yoga, meditation and the slow breathing techniques all mentioned in previous chapters are great tools to aid in relaxation. Two additional tools, sleep and massage, are discussed below.

SLEEP

Sleep is an essential component of overall health and well-being. Ensuring you have plenty of sleep and having that sleep be as deep and peaceful as possible will go a long way in supporting your mental, physical and emotional well-being. We live in a sleep-deprived society, where many people are not getting deep restorative sleep.[24] Too much light from cell phones, television, computers and other electronics contribute to constant stimulation and light hitting our eyes, which signals your body that it's still day time so that it takes longer to wind down. There are apps, like F.lux, that dim the light on your cell phones and computers as the sun goes down and for night time in order to help your body ease into rest more quickly after using those devices. You can also invest in blue-light-protecting glasses to reduce the strain on your eye from many hours of screen time. It's recommended that the best way to get a better night's rest is to turn off all electronics 15-30 min before going to bed to allow your body and mind to unwind and prepare for sleep. [25]

Sleep is vital for your physical health, as it is involved in the healing and repair of your heart and blood vessels.[26] Ongoing sleep deficiency is linked to an increased risk of heart disease, kidney disease, high blood pressure, diabetes, and stroke. If you are sleep deficient, you may have trouble making decisions, solving problems, controlling your emotions and behavior, and coping with change.[27] Sleep deficiency also has been linked to depression, suicide, and risk-taking behavior. The National Institute of Health (NIH) says sleep is vital to healthy brain function and emotional well-being, and that getting sufficient and quality sleep allows you to think clearly, make good decisions, manage your emotions, and respond, rather than react. [28]

MASSAGE

Anyone who has experienced the joy and pleasure of a good massage knows that it is a great way to reduce stress, eliminate toxins and relax both mind and body. Research shows that massage therapy relieves depression and anxiety by affecting the body's biochemistry.[29] Massage increases serotonin and dopamine, neurotransmitters that help reduce depression.[30] There are many types and styles of massage therapy, such as Swedish, deep tissue, Shiatsu, Thai, hot stone, and reflexology. Try exploring some of these and discover what you enjoy most and add massage therapy into your health routine. Search Yelp or search Massage in your App store and download a massage locator App.

ESSENTIAL OILS

To support you in sleeping better and enhance the massage experience and benefits, I recommend using pure therapeutic grade essential oils. Essential oils are natural extracts from the flowers, leaves, bark or root of plants. According to experts, aromatherapy from essential oils activates areas in your nose called smell receptors, which send messages through your nervous system to your brain.[31]

The oils activate certain areas of your brain, like your limbic system, which plays a role in your emotions and also has an impact on your hypothalamus, which responds to oils by creating feel-good brain chemicals like serotonin.[32]

Each oil has different properties and benefits, and many oils have calming, relaxing, and grounding effects. There are many oils that enhance relaxation of mind and body that you can add to your wellness routine and enjoy additional benefits. The seven best essential oils for anxiety, according to Dr. Axe, are lavender, rose, vetiver, Ylang Ylang, bergamot, frankincense, chamomile.[33]

It's important (and I've learned from experience) that not all oils are created equal and you want to ensure that you are using pure therapeutic grade essential oils that are sourced from flowers, plants and trees in their natural habitat and climate. You'll want to smell the oil and ensure it does not smell like alcohol or have a faint scent. It's also critical to ensure the pure oil is not mixed or diluted with a lesser oil. I have personally smelled oils that are clearly mixed with alcohol or a carrier oil.

I recommend using calming oils before bed. After turning off electronics 30 minutes before sleep to support you in winding down in the evening, Lavender is my go-to oil for calming and relaxing. Spraying a few drops on my pillow or putting a few drops in water in a diffuser fills the room and creates a great environment to rest and sleep peacefully.

Essential oils are also great to use topically during a massage to relax sore muscles. You can also use the oils as aromatherapy to relax your mind and body during the massage session. Try creating a calming, soothing atmosphere to relax your mind and body during your massage by asking your masseuse to add a few drops of your calming oil of choice to the headrest or diffusing it in the room.

TIP:

Try out one of the following Apps, such as:

- Sleep Cycle

- Slumber

- Relax Melodies: Sleep Solutions

- Relax Sounds

- Modern Essentials (essential oil information, recommendations, uses, etc.)

CHAPTER 11:
PRACTICE 6: HEALTHY EATING & DRINKING

In order to have your mind and body be well, it's vital that you nourish your body inside and out. Practice six is eating and drinking healthy. We've talked about the physical movement that you can do for your body; now let's explore how to fuel and nourish your body with food and drink. I'm not a nutritionist, and I don't pretend to know the best and healthiest foods for you. However, what I have learned over the years and during my own journey is that listening to your body is essential. We are often distracted by our racing minds and the busy world around us that we forget to listen to the most important person in one's life, yourself. You can tune in to notice when your body feels good and nourished while eating through your meditation and deep breathing practices.

As you expand your awareness and learn to be more present in the moment, you will begin listening to your body and noticing what sits well with you and what does not. Many people are not aware that they suffer from food sensitivities or intolerances because they fail to notice the signals their bodies send and then self-medicate to cover the signal. When they get an upset stomach or a headache, they take a pill. If they experience an itch on their skin, they rub on anti-itch lotion or take a pill. If they feel sluggish or tired after eating, they drink a caffeinated or sugar-full beverage, such as coffee or an energy drink. Through awareness, you can begin to notice what might be causing the discomfort before taking a pill. The pill will only relieve the symptom temporarily. How wonderful would it be if you could have the awareness to know what is healthy for you and begin to take less pills or take them less often? If you experience discomfort after eating, you can explore for yourself what you ate that may have caused that reaction. It may require eliminating one item at a time to determine which item, when eaten again, causes the same or similar reaction.

Psychiatrist Drew Ramsey says, "diet is potentially the most powerful intervention we have. By helping people shape their diets, we can improve their mental health and decrease their risk of psychiatric disorders." Recent studies have shown, "the risk of depression increases about 80% when you compare teens with a low-quality diet, or what we call the Western diet, to those who eat a higher-quality, whole-foods diet."[34] A whole-foods diet is food that is fresh or a diet rich in vegetables, fruits and whole grains, a whole food plant or seed in its natural form. The Western diet is mainly processed, packaged foods.

In today's fast-paced world, processed foods and snacks are easy and convenient, and as a result, the nutritional value of the typical standard American diet is greatly decreased.[35] Increasing your intake or ensuring you eat plenty of nutrient-rich fruits and vegetables, like leafy greens, can make a difference in your energy and how you feel. Part of a healthy diet is making sure you are drinking plenty of water to stay hydrated; pure water, in addition to or instead of juices, coffees and teas. These beverages contain water. However, they should not be relied on as the major source of your daily fluid intake. Another recommendation is lowering your sugar intake. One benefit of eating less sugar is that you will experience fewer hypoglycemic reactions such as sleepiness, hunger, and anxiety. Another benefit is a healthier weight. Sugar and refined carbs may contribute to obesity, regardless of the number of calories you take in.[36] Less sugar also improves heart health and supports healthier oral health and teeth.[37] Perhaps the best benefit, according to some dermatologists, is that less sugar can make you look younger because sugar breaks down the skin proteins, elastin and collagen. [38]

Here are some helpful reminders that you may have heard before. Eat mindfully; enjoy and savor your food and be aware of the experience. This will allow you to eat more slowly, which aids digestion and allows you to know when you are satisfied because your brain will have time to catch up with your body and send the signal that you are satisfied. Notice when you eat and feel satisfied, rather than full, and strive to eat until satisfied rather than full. Plan your meals ahead of time so that you are more in control of what you eat.

When I used to coach people regarding a specific diet protocol, one of the most important questions during the weekly check-in to assess progress would be whether or not they had daily bowel movements. Ensuring that your bodily waste is eliminated is essential to your health. Another important indicator of health and hydration is the color of your urine. A pale, straw color urine is best because this indicates you are well hydrated. We want all that does not serve us to flow out of us and be released physically for optimal well-being.

TIPS:

- Coffee and tea are diuretics and can dehydrate you. Stick to 8-12 oz per day to avoid dehydration.

- Drink ½ your body weight in ounces of water. Have a water bottle with clear oz marked on it and/or set up reminders to drink on Fitbit, on your phone or other device. Try the following Apps, WaterMinder, My Water Balance, or Daily Water Tracker Reminder

- Try the Whole 30 Diet

CHAPTER 12:
PRACTICE 7: GENEROSITY & GRATITUDE

Moving to the soul, the seventh and final practice is generosity and gratitude, and it starts with you. Are you grateful for who you are and what you have, little things and big things? Are you generous and loving with yourself? It's ok if you have not been. The question is: what are you choosing and creating, moving forward? Will you commit to being grateful each day for yourself, where you are and what you have? Will you commit to being your best friend, your biggest cheerleader and champion? Will you promise to be loving and generous with yourself, first and foremost?

Gratitude starts with being grateful for who you are, all that you have accomplished, all that you have, and all that you want for your future. Everyone, including you, has different gifts and talents. Your power, clarity and peace come from knowing yourself, your gifts and talents, and owning them, leveraging them, being grateful for them, celebrating them and sharing them with the world. If you are unsure of what they are, be curious, explore and discover what they might be. It's not about being perfect at something; it's about what you can contribute. You have a purpose; you matter. There is no need to compare yourself to others. Comparing brings negative energy based on false assumptions we make about others. We can never truly know what another person went through, gave up, had to do or become in order to accomplish and have what they have. Honor your uniqueness and the uniqueness of others. Honor yourself and be grateful for where you are now, the lessons you are learning and all you have in the present moment. There is always something you can be grateful for. Discover the little AND big things you can be grateful for and speak your gratitude out loud and write them down in your journal.

Building upon and sharing your gratitude brings us to generosity. In sharing your gratitude, you expand your generosity. Being generous starts with you being generous, loving and accepting to yourself. This is the foundation to be accepting of others and your circumstances. This state of generosity will allow you to experience greater peace and joy. Accepting does not mean you like the circumstances or situation. It does not mean putting up with things that do not support your well-being. Accepting means acknowledging that the situation, circumstance or person, including you, is the way it is. Resisting our past and current circumstances and situations prevents us from changing our future.

Generosity is sharing, sharing yourself and your gifts and being willing to receive and allow others to contribute to you as well. Research clearly demonstrates that improved social connection and support can improve mental health outcomes.[39] We are social beings. We are not meant to figure things out alone, to do it all alone, to face the world alone, to live our lives alone. You are not alone!! Be generous and vulnerable. Share what's really going on with you. Once you open up from a centered place, you will find there are many people eager, willing, and excited to support you. Being generous is allowing others the opportunity to provide support.

TIPS:

- Limit social media for 21 days. The temptation to compare to someone's highlight on social media can be a struggle. Try being grateful for their happiness and friendship.

- Make a gratitude list in your journal and pick one each day of the journey to focus on and deepen your connection – use the gratitude meditation on page 67 that item.

Clara V. Rodriguez

VIBRANT HAPPY YOU WORKBOOK

Now that you've finished the book, let's put it into practice to have you being healthy and happy. The following workbook is included to support you in creating an action plan to implement the practices daily until they become habits.

HOW TO GET THE MOST OUT OF THIS WORKBOOK

Each realm – mind, body and spirit – has practices, exercises, and suggestions for you to create your healthy mind, body and soul plan. Use the well-being tracker to log and keep track of your progress. By tracking in this way, you can see what realm needs more attention, celebrate what you have accomplished and ensure you have a balanced approach.

• • • VIBRANT HAPPY ME TRACKER • • •

		Mind		Body			Nutrition		Spirit	
Week of __/__/____		Meditation	Journal	Movement	Relaxation	Sleep	Water	Veggies	Generosity	Gratitude
Mon	Morning									
	Day									
	Night									
Tues	Morning									
	Day									
	Night									
Wed	Morning									
	Day									
	Night									
Thurs	Morning									
	Day									
	Night									
Fri	Morning									
	Day									
	Night									
Sat	Morning									
	Day									
	Night									
Sun	Morning									
	Day									
	Night									

PREPARATION FOR SUCCESS:

<u>Calendar</u>: To allow for success, it will be important to set aside dedicated time for each practice. Find a calendar system that will work for you to plan and schedule these activities. I recommend setting up reminders and/or alerts as needed to nudge you gently, to begin implementing these practices until they become regular habits.

<u>Support system</u>: Share what you are up to with people in your life, so they can support you in your well-being. Let them know you are committing to your wellness and that you will be meditating, making time for movement activities, rest and relaxation, and more. Maybe ask them to join you. Getting social will support you and make it fun.

<u>Journal or Notes place</u>: As you discover things you want to capture, you'll want to have your journal handy or an app on your phone to capture reflections, discoveries and awarenesses.

<u>Suggestion</u>: Journal for 5 minutes a day

<u>Celebrate</u>: Make time to celebrate at the end of each week. Honoring and acknowledging yourself for all that you have accomplished each day and week is a part of your generosity and gratitude practice.

<u>Suggestion</u>s: Take a Bath or a nice walk, read a book you enjoy or watch a movie, rather than eating pie, cake, a whole pizza or bag of chips, drinking, or other habits you are letting go of.

AWARENESS OF MIND

STEP: 1: IDENTIFYING YOUR LIMITING BELIEFS

Before we get into practical examples for turning each practice into a habit, let's begin by identifying your limiting beliefs. This is yours, so be straight and honest with yourself. That is the access to shifting your mind. This exercise should take ~ 20 minutes, plus follow-up time.

What's your story? What do you tell yourself over and over again that might be contributing to you being anxious or depressed?

_____

_____

_____

_____

Rewrite your story. Who do you want to create yourself as? Who and how do you want to be? First, close your eyes and visualize it, then write it down.

_____

_____

_____

_____

Make a commitment to yourself to be/live into that new story. What is one action that you can take to fulfill on that commitment to have it be your new story? put it on your calendar.

_____

_____

_____

_____

What is the exact situation, when will you do this action, when will you take this action, how will it look?

_____

_____

_____

_____

Share your new story with someone. Write down 1-3 people you will call and share your new story with. Then, take out your calendar (paper or electronic) and schedule the time to make the calls to share.

_____

_____

_____

_____

Rather than figuring out the why, to better understand yourself, ask what. What are the situations that make me feel sad or anxious?

_____

_____

_____

_____

What do they have in common?

_____

_____

_____

_____

What are some things I can do right now to feel better and support my well-being?

_____

_____

_____

_____

What should I do next to move my desire for a vibrant, happy me forward?

_____

_____

_____

_____

Who can support me in moving this forward?

_____

_____

_____

_____

What do I need to learn or know to move this forward?

_____

_____

_____

_____

AWARENESS OF MIND

PRACTICE 1 – MEDITATION

Let's begin the journey and explore what the best meditation technique for your 21-day journey is.

To make meditation a habit and receive the full benefits, meditate 15 minutes a day, every day, consistently. The first week, you can ease into it starting the first two days with five minutes, next two days, ten minutes each, and by the fifth day, beginning 15 minutes of meditation. Or feel free to dive right in and meditate for 15 minutes a day. Included here are a few different types of meditations. For more meditations, check out my website: www.clarav.com

Meditation Focus Breath ~ 15 min

Find a comfortable place to sit where you will not be disturbed for 10-15 minutes. If you are sitting in a chair, place your feet on the floor and sit up tall, relax your shoulders. If your feet don't touch the floor, try placing a pillow on the floor to have them rest comfortably. If you are seated in your bed or on the floor, sit up tall and relax your shoulders. The most important thing here is to be comfortable. Close your eyes and begin to go inward, breathing deeply. Focus on your breath. As thoughts arise, simply notice them, become an observer and then let them go. Come back to your breath, inhaling deeply, expanding the belly, exhaling completely, bringing your awareness to the present moment. As thoughts continue to come in, notice them and let go. Continue bringing your focus back to your breath, inhaling and exhaling deeply.

Helpful tools resources

Insight Timer App – allows you to listen to calming sounds while you meditate, and has the option to sound a gong, chime, or other sounds at intervals to help remind you to focus back on your mantra or breath. My personal favorite is to set a 15-minute timer with five-minute interval bells and moonlight ambient sound with a different ending bell to let you know the 15 minutes have elapsed.

Meditation Focus Mantra ~15 min

Find a comfortable place to sit where you will not be disturbed for 10-15 minutes. Place your feet on the floor, or have your legs comfortably crossed or extended and sit up tall, relax your shoulders. Close your eyes and begin to go inward, breathing deeply. Begin incorporating the mantra, So Hum. On your inhale, silently in your mind, say, "So." On the exhale, silently in your mind, say, "Hum." On each inhale, repeat "So," and on each exhale, "Hum." As thoughts arise, let them float away and keep bringing yourself back to gently repeating the mantra – So, Hum. Continue relaxing and repeating the mantra, "So Hum" as you inhale and exhale deeply. Continuing bringing your focus back to the mantra, inhaling and exhaling deeply.

Gratitude Meditation ~15 min

Sit comfortably, close your eyes, and take several slow, deep breaths. Inhaling deeply through the nose, exhaling, relaxing, breathing out through the nose. Take a couple of deep breaths with your eyes closed and spend a few minutes thinking of each of the following, while continuing to breathe deeply.

Think of something good that has happened to you recently.

Think of someone you love, appreciate, and are happy to have in your life.

Think of an occasion when you were honored or appreciated by others.

Think about what you are grateful for about your present situation and what is going on in your life.

PRACTICE 2 – DECLARATION

Building upon your new story: visualize who you want to be and how you want to be. Who do you want to declare yourself as today? Now, write it down here or in your journal.

Who I am is _____

I am _____

SOME SUGGESTIONS:

powerful	happy	free
kind	loving	generous
peaceful	calm	joyful
carefree	positive	Friendly

Exercise:

Stand up in front of a mirror. Look at the beautiful human being looking back at you, and smile. Look yourself straight in the eyes, and with a huge smile, declare out loud to yourself and the world exactly who and how you want to be.

AWARENESS OF BODY

Notice how you are sitting right now. Are you hunched over, is your back rounded? How is your breathing? Is it shallow? Do your shoulders rise when you inhale or is your breathe deep originating in the low belly?

Notice your body – notice your neck, shoulders, scan from head to toe.

Notice and release – Let go, relax, exhale.

PRACTICE 3 – DEEP BREATHING

Deep breathing is a simple practice to add in daily. In the well-being tracker, it is listed in the relaxation section. However, you can use deep breathing to start off your day, end your day, or any time get you back to calmness. You can easily add this to the beginning of your meditation routine to prepare you for meditation.

Exercise:

Sit up tall with a straight back. Bring both hands to your belly. Relax your shoulders. Inhale deeply through your nose, filling your diaphragm with air completely, expanding your belly like a balloon. On the exhale, continue to relax deeply, slowly releasing all the air from your belly, bringing your navel towards your spine. Inhale deeply, expanding your belly completely, notice your chest and ensure you are breathing from your diaphragm rather than your chest. To ensure you are breathing from your diagram, notice your regular breath. Then, drop your inhale as low as you can. Can you feel it below your belly button and deep into your lower back? Perhaps, you can feel your inhale all the way down to your pelvic floor. Continue focusing on your breath and the expansion and contraction of your belly.

PRACTICE 4 – MOVEMENT

Think about what activities you enjoy or want to explore as part of your movement routine. Do you enjoy yoga, exercise, Zumba, hiking, running, and/or biking? Make a list of the activities you will commit to incorporating into your wellness routine on a regular basis. Use the first letter of each to trail on your well-being tracker.

_____

_____

_____

_____

To set yourself up for success, in addition to scheduling time for your movement activities, asking someone to join you or finding a group activity that has you moving, find ways to make it easy to get up and get moving. Some suggestions are to sleep in your workout clothes or leave them next to the bed, sign up for a gym or class, and/or find someone to hold you accountable to get moving on the days and times you set on your calendar.

TIP:

Go to a running store for running groups or visit Meetup.com for hiking, yoga, or other fitness activity group

YOGA

Incorporate these yoga poses along with deep breathing into your daily morning or evening routine.

CHILD POSE – BALASANA

It's a gentle resting pose that stretches the hips, thighs and legs, while calming the mind and relieving stress and tension.

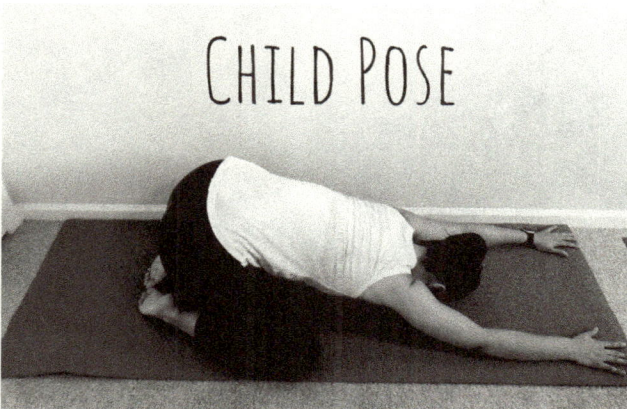

CHILD POSE

CHILD POSE INSTRUCTIONS:

- Begin on hands and knees

- Knees can be wide to the edge of the mat or together

- Press your hips back toward your heels, moving your seat toward your feet

- Lengthen your arms out in front of you

- Rest your forehead onto the floor (or pillow, or block)

- Begin connecting with your breath

- Deep inhales through the nose, expanding the belly into the thighs

- Full exhalation breathing out the low back

RECLINED BOUND ANGLE POSE – SUPTA BADAKONSANA

Helps relieve symptoms of stress, anxiety, and depression.

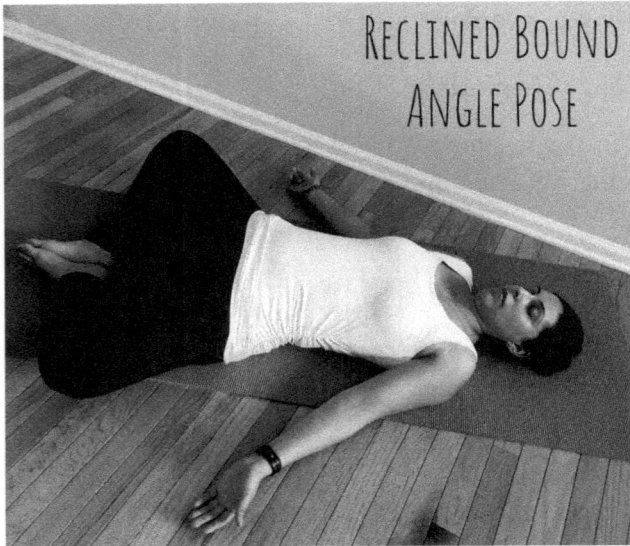

RECLINED BOUND ANGLE POSE INSTRUCTIONS:

- Begin laying on your back

- Bend your knees and bring the soles of your feet together to touch, letting your knees fall out wide towards the edges of the mat – use pillows or blocks under knees for added comfort

- Lengthen your tailbone to create a long, low back

- Bring shoulders away from your ears and allow arms to rest along the sides of your body, palms face up

- Relax head, neck and jaw

- Breathe deeply, inhaling filling the belly completely, expanding it like a balloon, on the exhale, relax the entire body a little more, letting the knees relax towards the floor and bring the navel towards the floor

- Continue inhaling and exhaling deeply, starting and ending at the low belly

LEGS UP THE WALL POSE – VIPARITA KARANI

Legs up the wall is a gentle inversion that calms the mind and eases anxiety and stress. This pose can help practice the art of surrender.

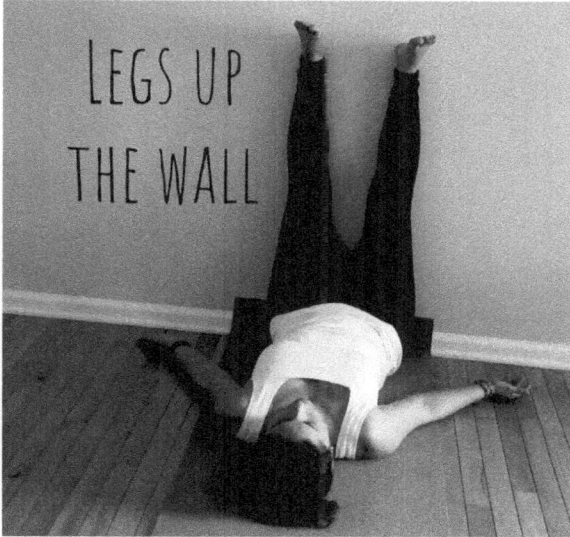

LEGS UP THE WALL INSTRUCTIONS:

- To begin, sit right up next to the wall with one hip touching the wall. (If an empty wall is not accessible, you can place a yoga block under the sacrum or the flat part of your low back and bring your legs up in the air.)

- Bring your right hand to the floor next to you to support you, and on your exhale, gently swing your legs up against the wall, while you bring your back, shoulders and head to rest on the floor.

- Keep your chin neutral, rather than tucked in towards your chest. Let the back of your neck lie flat.

- Open your shoulder blades away from the spine and release your arms and hands out to your side, palms up. Soften and close your eyes and take several deep breaths.

- To exit, bend your knees and bring the soles of your feet against the wall.

- Rest here a few breaths, then roll onto your side. Lie on your side for a few breaths, make sure to get up slowly. Getting up too fast can result in lightheadedness.

WIDE-LEGGED STANDING FORWARD FOLD
– PRASARITA PADOTTANASANA

Is a calming forward bend. It calms the mind, provides relief to stress, anxiety and mild depression. It quiets and soothes the nervous system.

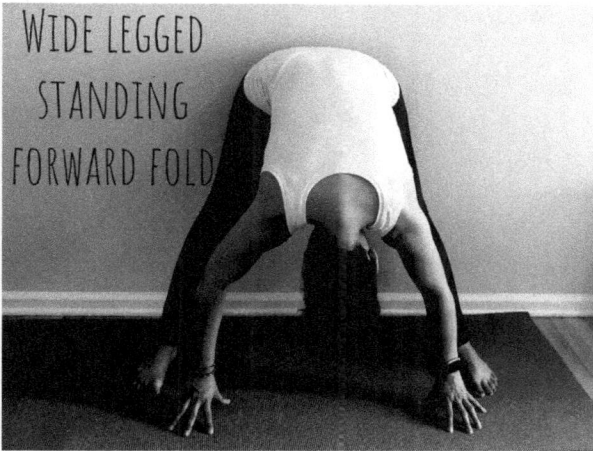

WIDE-LEGGED STANDING FORWARD FOLD INSTRUCTIONS:

- To begin, start by standing tall at the front of your mat

- Bring your hands to your hips, turn to the left and step your feet wide apart

- Turn your toes slightly in and your heels slightly out, and align your heels

- Inhale and lengthen your torso, reaching through the crown of your head

- Exhale, fold forward at the hips

- Drop your head and gaze softly behind you

- If your head does not come to the floor, you can rest it on yoga block(s)

- Continue breathing deeply here for several deep breaths, relaxing more deeply with each exhale

- To release, bring your hands to your hips. Press firmly through your feet, inhale to lift your torso, while maintaining a flat back.

PRACTICE 5 – RELAXATION

Think about what activities relaxes you. Does painting, reading, listening to music, massage, taking a walk, going for a gentle hike and/or getting a facial relax you? Make a list of the activities you will commit to incorporating into your wellness routine on a regular basis.

I will choose from the following activities regularly to ensure relaxation is part of my weekly routine.

_____

_____

_____

_____

Explore therapeutic grade essential oils and see what oils soothe, calm and relax you. Use oils as part of your bedtime routine. Try lavender on your pillow or diffuse lavender in your bedroom at night.

PRACTICE 6 – HEALTHY EATING AND DRINKING

When you feel hungry, ask yourself, "What am I really hungry for or in need of at this moment? Is it really food I am needing?"

Are you eating to satisfy some unmet need or emotion?

Exercise: Eat more slowly and mindfully, savor each bite, see if you can notice when you feel satisfied and put down the fork or spoon and enjoy the feeling of satisfaction and be complete with your meal. Use the Chocolate Meditation below to experience mindful eating and see how you can take what you discover and apply it to all your meals and snacks.

Exercise: Chocolate Meditation

1. Start with a small piece of chocolate: I recommend a small piece of dark chocolate, 60% plus cocoa content, but you can use a chocolate kiss, a handful of semi-sweet chips, or whatever you have on-hand. Bite-sized or a little larger is best.

2. Begin relaxing your body: Take a few deep breaths and untense all the muscles in your body to relax your entire body. Close your eyes. You want to be as relaxed as possible.

3. Smell, nibble and savor: Smell the chocolate and enjoy the aroma. Take a small bite of your chocolate. Let it sit on your tongue and melt in your mouth. Notice the flavors from the chocolate, become completely absorbed in what you are experiencing. Continue your deep breathing, and concentrate on the sensations in your mouth, noticing each and every one.

4. Focus on sensations: As you swallow, focus on how it feels going down. Notice how your mouth feels empty. Then, as you take a second bite, try to even notice how your arm feels as you raise the chocolate to your mouth, how it feels between your fingers, and then in your mouth. Again, focus on the sensations you are feeling in the present moment.

5. Re-focus on the present: If other thoughts come into your mind during your chocolate meditation, gently refocus your attention to the flavors and sensations associated with the chocolate. The idea is to stay in the present moment as much as possible.

6. Savor this feeling: When you are done savoring your chocolate, revisit the feeling throughout your day, and feel more relaxed.

TIPS:

You don't need to consume large quantities of chocolate during this exercise. In fact, if you're doing it carefully, you won't need to consume much at all.

If you're sensitive to chocolate or have issues with sugar, you can try a similar type of meditation with a grape, small fruit or other savorable food you are able to eat.

Set yourself up for success:

Have water on the nightstand for your morning routine. Prep food at night or on weekends to have healthy snack options during the day. Nuts, celery sticks, cucumber sticks or slices, and carrots are good options.

TIP:

To ensure you get your leafy greens in, consider making a healthy, low sugar smoothie as part of your morning routine. Here's a simple recipe:

- 6 cups leafy greens (ex: kale, spinach, chard or other greens)

- 1 banana or ⅓ cup fruit frozen (if not frozen, add five ice cubes)

- ¾ cup sugar-free/no-sugar-added nut milk of choice or water

- ¼ cup of flax or chia seeds

- Blend on high until smooth

PRACTICE 7 – GENEROSITY AND GRATITUDE

Make time and be intentional to share something with someone throughout your day. Share a smile, a hug, a meal, a laugh. Share about your weekend, your day, or your plans. Get social and make time to share something with someone. Be generous with your time, your listening, and yourself.

Discover ways to be grateful in each moment. If you find yourself reacting to circumstances and events around you, catch yourself or simply notice, take a deep breath and shift your perspective by asking yourself the following questions.

- "What's good about this?"

- "What can I learn from this?"

- "How can I benefit from this?"

- "Is there something about this situation that I can be grateful for?"

Create a list of 100 things that you are grateful for. If it helps, divide your list into different categories, such as assets (things you own), people (your relationships), qualities (personal qualities and character traits), experiences (places you've visited and things you've done), and so on.

Morning Gratitude:

Each morning before stepping out of bed, with your eyes open or closed, say out loud or in your head – THANK YOU! Thank you for this day, thank you for my life. Choose a few more things to be grateful for and start your day with gratitude.

Bedtime Gratitude:

Before going to bed each night, write a list of five things about that day for which you are grateful. Some days you'll have exciting things to write down, and some days you'll be writing down simple joys. Both are perfect and wonderful. Let a smile be the last thing you do. Say thank you to the universe and sleep sweetly.

MEET THE ARTISTS

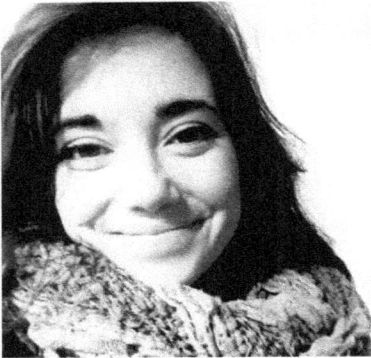

Ilana Rose Cloud is an artist, a freelance web designer and graphic designer living in Portland, OR. She has been making art in one form or another since she was three years old, having found from an early age that creating gives her space to focus, calm, and ground.

She continues to use her art practice as a way to reduce stress and cultivate peace.

Ilana has a Bachelor of Fine Arts in Painting and Printmaking. Artistic spirit and energy weaves its way throughout her life and is currently propelling her towards a long-time dream of pursuing a master's in Naturopathic Medicine and Acupuncture.

Ilana works with clients all over the country to strengthen their brand, reinvigorate their online presence, or invent the image of a new business. You can find her design portfolio at www.cloudsparkdesigns.com and her artwork at www.ilanarosecloud.com.

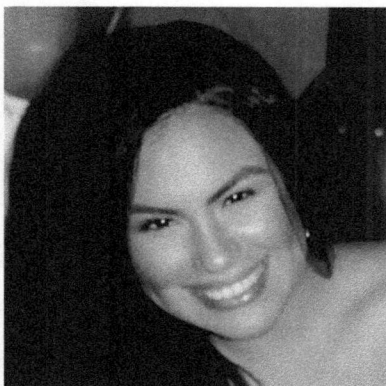

During her high school and college years, Samantha has been involved with numerous non-profit organizations. After graduating from college with a degree in Non-profit Administration, she continued to do so. Making a difference in the community while capturing priceless moments along the way.

Since a young age, Samantha has always been drawn to taking photos. She finds great passion and joy in being able to bring to life special moments and capturing moments of a community coming together, celebrations and festivities. Her work often serves to raise awareness in the hope of igniting change. Partnering with nonprofits has given Samantha the opportunity to connect with beautiful people and allow them to share their story.

In her free time, Samantha enjoys being outdoors, spending time with family, and of course, snapping photos along the way.

Instagram: samleexo

YOUR "task" IS NOT
TO SEEK love BUT MERELY TO
SEEK AND find
ALL THE barriers WITHIN
yourself THAT YOU HAVE
BUILT against IT.

RUMI

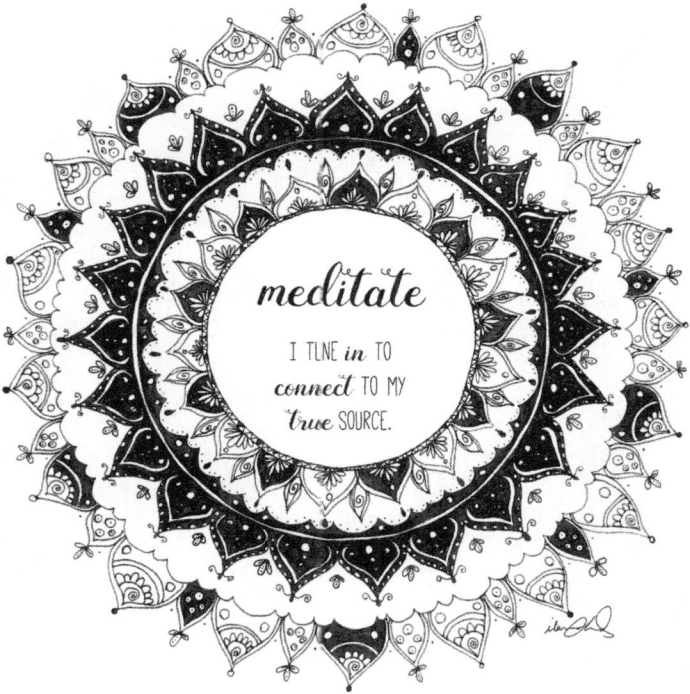

meditate

I TUNE *in* TO
connect TO MY
true SOURCE.

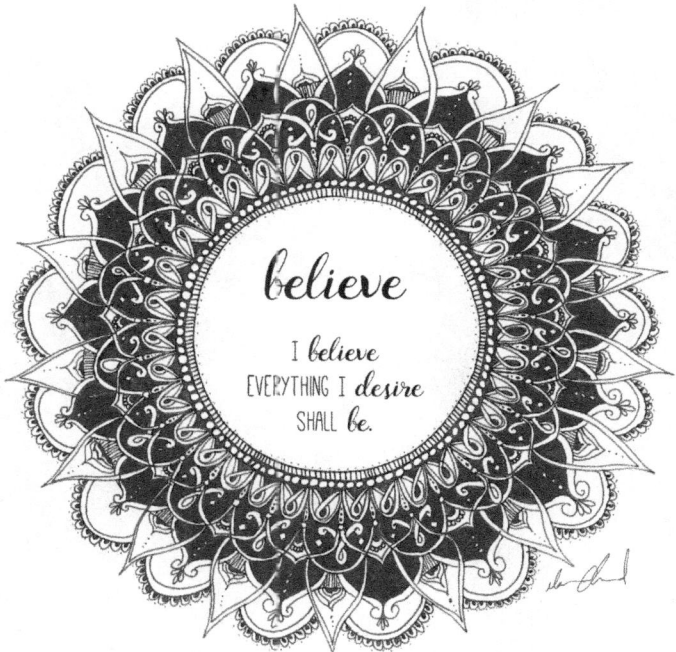

believe

I believe
EVERYTHING I desire
SHALL be.

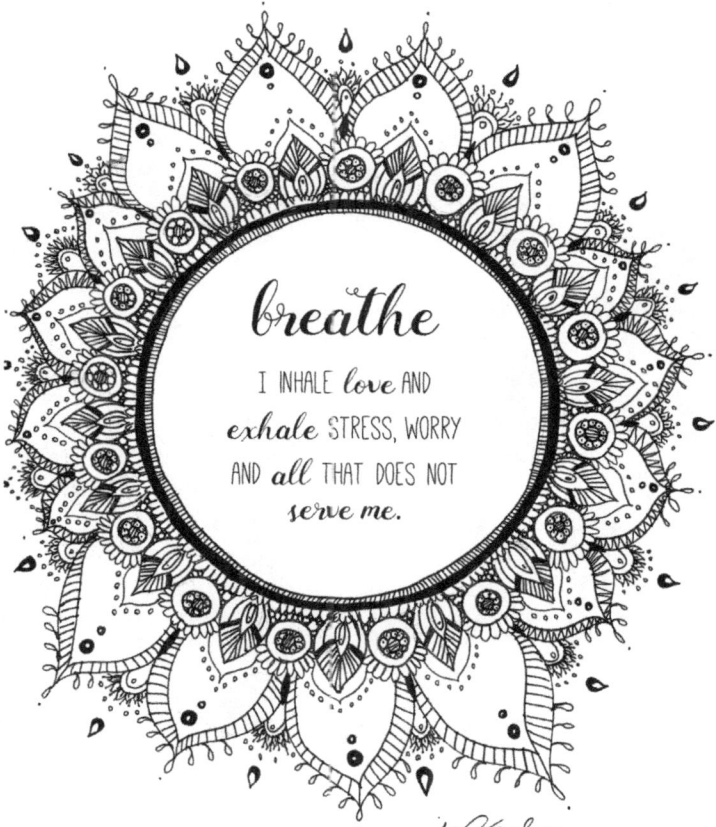

breathe

I INHALE *love* AND
exhale STRESS, WORRY
AND *all* THAT DOES NOT
serve me.

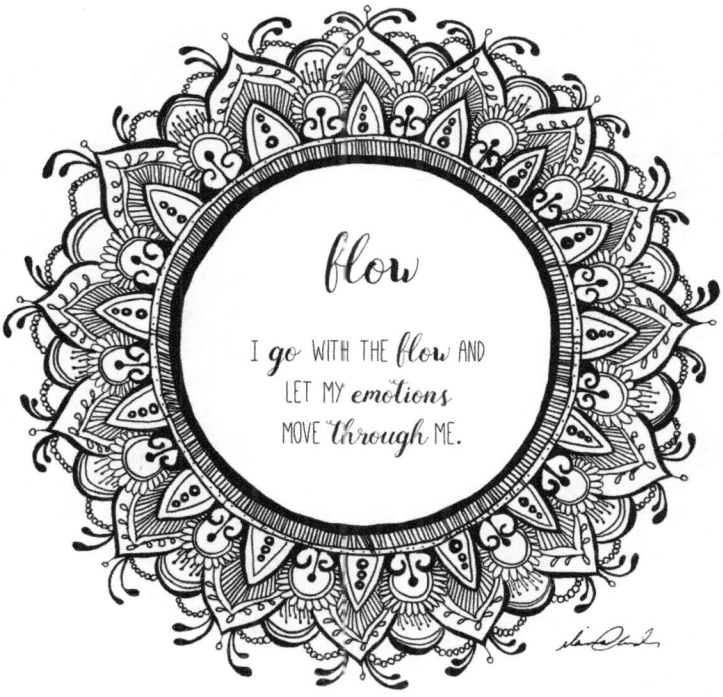

flow

I go WITH THE *flow* AND
LET MY *emotions*
MOVE *through* ME.

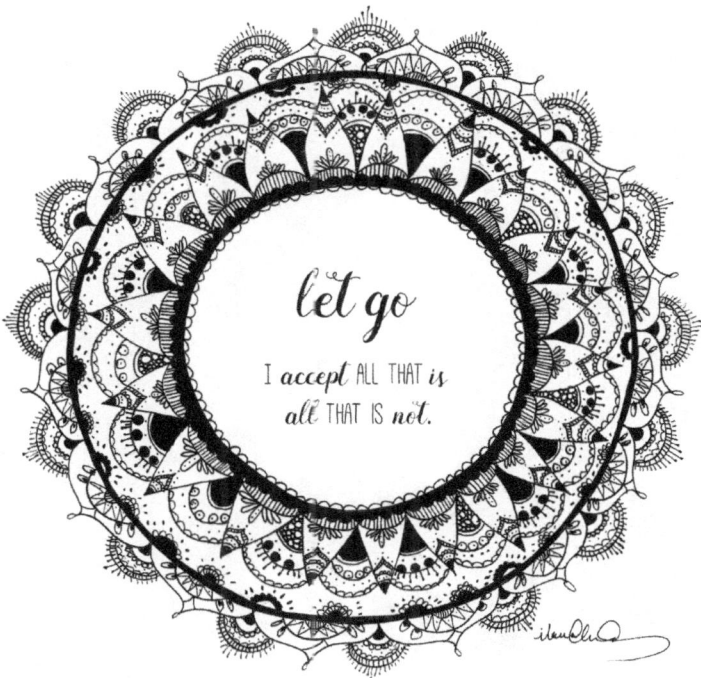

let go

I accept ALL THAT *is*
all THAT IS *not*.

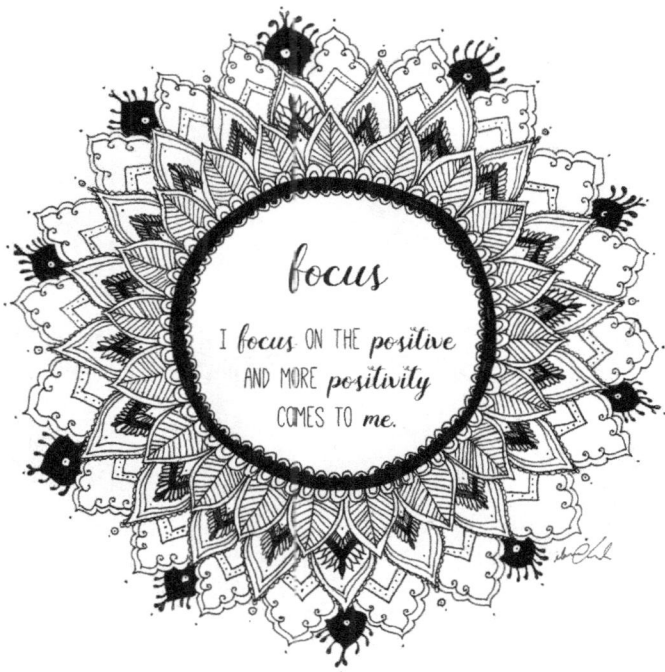

focus

I focus ON THE positive
AND MORE positivity
COMES TO me.

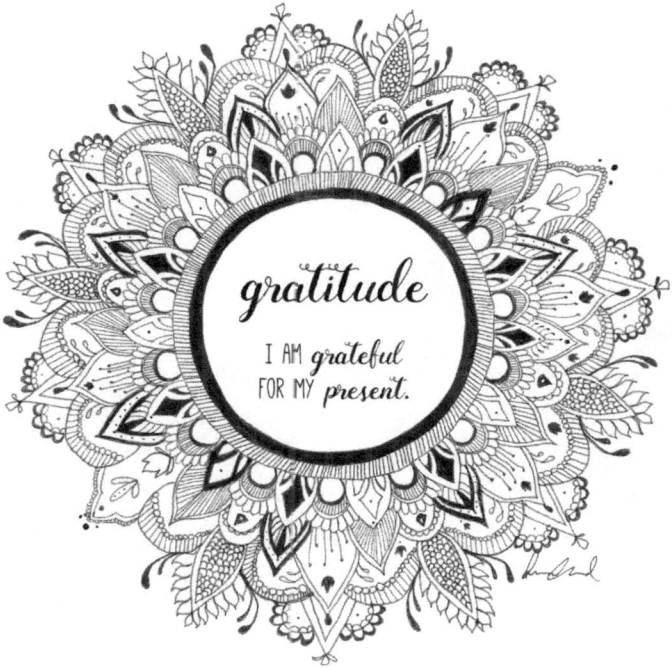

gratitude

I AM *grateful*
FOR MY *present*.

BIBLIOGRAPHY

For viewable link, visit: www.clarav.com/vhy-resources/

1. Can What You Eat Affect Your Mental Health? Kelli Miller – WebMD

2. Nearly 1 in 5 Americans Suffers From Mental Illness Each Year.

Victoria Bekiempis – Newsweek

3. Depression: 'Second Biggest Cause Of Disability' in World

Helen Briggs – BBC News

4. Can What You Eat Affect Your Mental Health? Kelli Miller – WebMD

5. Meditation: In Depth, NCCIH

6. Mind the Mat, 200-Hour Yoga Teacher Training Manual, 2014

7. Embodied Cognition, Robert Wilson-Lucia Foglia

8. The Surprising And Powerful Links Between Posture and Mood

Vivian Giang – FastCompany

9. There's Magic in Your Smile: How Smiling Affects Your Brain – Ronald E Riggio, Ph.D. Psychology Today

10, 11. Breathing For Life: The Mind-body Healing Benefits Of Pranayama, Sheila Patel, M.D.

12. Anxiety Always Comes With Shallow Breathing – Calm Clinic

13. Exercise and Depression – WebMD

14. Endorphins and Exercise, V Harber-J Sutton – NIH

15. Why Does Your Body Release Endorphins While You're Exercising? | Healthfully – LiveStrong

16, 17. How Simply Moving Benefits Your Mental Health

Srini Pillay – Harvard

18. Effects Of Dance Movement Therapy and Dance on Health-related Psychological Outcomes: A Meta-analysis

Sabine Koch PhD, Teresa Kunz M.Sc., Sissy Lykou MA, Robyn Cruz PhD – Scientist Direct

19. Effects of Music Therapy Strategy on Depressed Older Adults

Hanser SB1, Thompson LW.

20, 21. Does Music Have Healing Powers? Michael Friedman Ph.D. – Psychology Today

22. Relaxation Techniques: Try These Steps To Reduce Stress, Mayo Clinic Staff

23. Relaxation Training For Anxiety: A Ten-year Systematic Review with Meta-analysis, Gian Mauro Manzoni, Francesco Pagnini, Gianluca Castelnuovo, Enrico Molinari

24, 26, 27. The Toll Of Sleep Loss in America, Jeanie Davis – WebMD

25. Power Down for Better Sleep, Heather Hatfield – WebMD

28. The Benefits Of Slumber: Why You Need a Good Night's Sleep. HIH News in Health, April 2003

29, 30. Massage a Powerful tool to fight depression and anxiety naturally, Mara Nicandro LMT, NMT, MMT, NKT®, HLC1

31, 32. What Is Aromatherapy? – WebMD

33. The Top 7 Essential Oils For Anxiety, Dr. Axe

34, 35. Can What You Eat Affect Your Mental Health? Kelli Miller – WebMD

36, 37, 38. What Are the Benefits Of Lowering Your Sugar Intake? Virginia Vynckt

39. Social Ties and Mental Health Ichiro Kawachi, Lisa Berkman – NIH

www.ingramcontent.com/pod-product-compliance
Lightning Source LLC
Chambersburg PA
CBHW030258030426
42336CB00009B/431